B.L. Bauer and T.J. Kuhn (Eds.), Severe Head Injuries

Springer
Berlin
Heidelberg
New York
Barcelona
Budapest
Hong Kong
London
Milan
Paris
Santa Clara
Singapore
Tokyo

B.L. Bauer and T.J. Kuhn (Eds.)

Severe Head Injuries

Pathology, Diagnosis and Treatment

With 15 Figures and 6 Tables

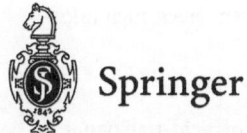 Springer

Prof. Dr. med. Bernhard L. Bauer
Dr. med. Thomas J. Kuhn
Philipps-Universität Marburg
Zentrum für Operative Medizin I
Baldingerstraße
D-35043 Marburg

ISBN-13: 978-3-642-64544-0   Springer-Verlag Berlin Heidelberg

Cataloging-in-Publication Data applied for
Die Deutsche Bibliothek – CIP-Einheitsaufnahme

Severe head injuries : pathology, diagnosis and treatment ; with 6 tables /
B. L. Bauer and T. J. Kuhn (ed.) – Berlin ; Heidelberg ; New York ; Barcelona ;
Budapest ; Hong Kong ; London ; Milan ; Paris ; Santa Clara ; Singapore ;
Tokyo : Springer 1997
ISBN-13: 978-3-642-64544-0   eISBN-13: 978-3-642-60761-5
DOI:10.1007/978-3-642-60761-5

© Springer-Verlag Berlin Heidelberg 1997
Softcover reprint of the hardcover 1st edition 1997

Cover Design: E. Kirchner, Heidelberg
Typesetting: FotoSatz Pfeifer GmbH, Gräfelfing
SPIN: 10556469   81/3135 – 5 4 3 2 1 0 – Printed on acid-free paper

Preface

The management of severely brain-injured patients is one of the special obligations of the neurosurgeon. The outcome – on the other hand – depends on a multidisciplinary, integrated approach among all the specialists involved.

Two hundred years ago, Alexander Monro, the Scottish anatomist, started conducting research on pathological changes following head injury. This book covers different aspects of neurotraumatology up to the end of this century.

The surgical and medical treatment of severely brain-injured patients continues to present a challenge to neurosurgeons. We would like to express our gratitude to our colleagues for contributing outstanding presentations of their research and clinical experience to this book. The past decade has seen tremendous advances in areas such as magnetic resonance, transcranial Doppler ultrasound, critical care medicine, multimodal monitoring, and special brain tissue pO_2 measurements concurrent with ICP. These have greatly added to our ability to understand the natural history of brain damage and also contributed to the successful treatment of severely brain-injured patients.

The purpose of the present volume is to reflect the current state of theoretical research and to provide support for daily bedside practice. We admit that we cannot present the entire spectrum of knowledge associated with the pathophysiology of brain injury in one reference book and thus invite any further discussion or criticism.

Finally, our thanks are extended to all contributors for meeting the deadlines and to our ever-patient editor at Springer, Agnes Heinz, who must be thanked for shepharding this project from its inception to its completion.

B.L. Bauer   T.J. Kuhn

Contents

1 Clinical Head Injury Trials
R. Braakman   1

2 Pathophysiology of Brain Injury
T.J. Kuhn   6

3 The Morphology of Traumatic Head Injury: An Overview
H.D. Mennel   19

4 Preclinical Emergency Management of Severe Brain Injuries and Polytraumata
P. Sefrin and C. Apfel   29

5 Preclinical Treatment of Patients With Severe Brain Injuries
J. Piek   34

6 The Traumatic Carotid Cavernous Fistula:
Clinical Features, Diagnosis, and Therapy
S. Bien and J.P. Wakat   44

7 Guidelines for the Management of Severe Head Injury:
An Overview
R.M. Chesnut   50

8 Cranial Fractures and Traumatic Hematomas
R. Firsching   68

9 Panfacial Fractures
W. Hochban   76

10 Cerebral Blood Flow, Hyperventilation, and Metabolism in
Severe Head Injury
D.W. Marion   82

11 Management of Intracranial Hypertension in Pediatric
Head Injury
M.J. Fritsch, K.H. Manwaring, and D.H. Beyda   89

12 Quality and Therapeutic Advances in Multimodality
Neuromonitoring Following Head Injury
*J. Meixensberger, A. Jäger, J. Dings, S. Baunach,
and K. Roosen* 99

13 Monitoring of Cerebral Oxygenation in Traumatic Brain
Injured Patients
*A.S. Sarrafzadeh, A.W. Unterberg, K.L.Kiening, T.F. Bardt,
G.-H. Schneider, and W.R. Lanksch* 109

14 Traumatic Lesions of Cranial Nerves in Head-Injured
Patients
M. Samii and C. Matthies 121

15 Neurological, Neurophysiological Syndromes and Cognitive
Disorders in Brain-Injured Patients: Epidemiology, Diagnosis,
and Therapeutic Advances
W. Gobiet 142

Subject Index 151

List of Contributors

Bien, Siegfried, Prof. Dr., Leiter der Abt. für Neuroradiologie, MZ für Nervenheilkunde
Rudolf-Bultmann-Straße 8, 35039 Marburg, Germany
Tel. (06421) 28-6255, Fax (06421) 28-8967

Chesnut, Randall M., M.D., Director of Neurotrauma and Neurosurgical Critical Care, Oregon Health Sciences University, School of Medicine, Division of Neurosurgery
3181 S.W. Sam Jackson Park Road, Portland, OR 97201-3098, USA
Tel. 001 503 494-8070, Fax 001 503 494 7161

Firsching, Raimund, Prof. Dr., Direktor der Neurochirurgischen Universitätsklinik, Otto v. Guericke-Universität
Leipziger Straße 44, 39120 Magdeburg, Germany
Tel. (0391) 671-55334, Fax (0391) 671-5544

Gobiet, Wolfgang, Dr., Ärztlicher Direktor der Neurologischen Klinik, Postfach 280, 31810 Hess. Oldendorf, Germany
Tel. (05152) 781-231, Fax (05152) 781-198

Hochban, Walter, PD Dr. Dr., Oberarzt der Klinik für Mund-, Kiefer- und Gesichtschirurgie
Georg-Voigt-Straße 3, 35039 Marburg, Germany
Tel. (06421) 28-3209, Fax (06421) 28-8990

Kuhn, Thomas J., Dr., Klinik für Neurochirurgie, Philipps-Universität, Baldingerstraße, 35033 Marburg, Germany
Tel. (06421) 28-3237, Fax (06421) 28-5751

Manwaring, Kim, M.D., Director, Pediatric Neurosurgery, Phoenix Children's Hospital, 909 East Brill Street
Phoenix, Arizona 85006, USA
Tel.: 001 602 496 8270, FAX 001 602 254 7202

Marion, Donald W., M.D., Associate Professor of Neurological Surgery, Suite B 400, Presbyterian University Hospital
200 Lothrop Street, Pittsburgh, PA 15213-2582, USA
Tel. 001 412 647-5559

Mennel, Hans Dieter, Prof. Dr., Leiter des Institutes für Neuro-
pathologie, MZ für Pathologie, Baldingerstraße, 35033 Marburg
Tel. (06421) 28-2282, Fax (06421) 28-5640

Meixensberger, Jürgen, PD Dr., Oberarzt der Neurochirurgischen
Univ.-Klinik, Josef-Schneider-Straße 11, 97080 Würzburg
Tel. (0931) 201 5800, Fax (0931) 201 2635

Piek, Jürgen, Prof. Dr., Oberarzt der Neurochirurgischen Univ.-
Klinik, Ernst-Moritz-Arndt-Universität
Sauerbruchstraße, 17489 Greifwald
Tel. (3834) 86-6162, Fax (03834) 86-6164

Samii, Madjid, Prof. Dr. Dr., Direktor der Neurochirurgischen
Klinik der Medizinischen Hochschule, Direktor der Neurochirur-
gischen Klinik/Krankenhaus Nordstadt
Haltenhoffstraße 41, 30167 Hannover
Tel. (0511) 970-1245, Fax (0511) 970-1606

Sefrin, Peter, Prof. Dr., Leiter der Notfallmedizinischen Abteilung
der Universität Würzburg, Josef-Schneider-Straße 11
97080 Würzburg

Unterberg, Andreas, Prof. Dr., Oberarzt der Neurochirurgischen
Klinik, Virchow-Klinikum, Humboldt-Universität zu Berlin
Augustenburger Platz 1, 13353 Berlin
Tel. (030) 45060-001, Fax (030) 45060-900

1 Clinical Head Injury Trials

R. Braakman

During the last decade, outcome in severely head-injured patients has improved due to changes in management regimens, better organization, introduction of guidelines in various countries [1, 2], founding of the American and European Brain Injury Consortia (ABIC and EBIC), and other factors. Altered pharmacotherapy is one of these.

Attempts to ameliorate the negative effects of secondary brain damage by pharmacotherapy require clinical trials. Pharmaceutical agents believed to have a favorable effect are first tested in dose-escalating studies with regard to bioavailability, pharmacokinetics, and drug safety in phase 1 trials in healthy individuals. Subsequently, in phase 2 trials the drug's safety and, on a limited scale, effectivity are assessed in small groups of patients:

- Phase 1
  Drug safety
  Human volunteers
  Dose escalation experiments
- Phase 2
  Targeted population (patients)
  Efficacy and safety
  Small scale

These phase 1 and 2 trials result in many drugs being discarded because of side effects. Pharmacists of large companies tell that about 10 % of drugs pass through this sieve. The effectivity of the remainder is assessed by subjecting them to full-scale phase three randomized placebo-controlled trials:

- Phase 3
  Full-scale evolution of efficacy
- Phase 4
  Postmarketing surveillance of adverse effects

In these studies two types of error must be taken into account:

- Type 1 (alpha) error: indicator of a false positive effect – the treatment seems to be beneficial, but it is not better than control
- Type 2 (or beta error): indicator of a false negative effect – the treatment seems to be not beneficial, but in fact it is better than control; power is 1 minus beta.

It is considered to be highly unlikely that in severe head injury a drug dimi-
nishes a bad outcome by more than 5 %. In most trials a type 1 error of 5 % and
a power of 80 % – 90 % are considered to be optimal. Phase 3 trials should
therefore include well over 800 patients, something which is only possible in
international, multicenter trials. It is obvious that such large trials, involving
enormous costs, are feasible only with the finantial support of pharmaceutical
companies or other sponsors.

The results of some of the trials on head injury that have been published in
the literature, or which are currently underway and of interest to clinicians are
reported. We should be aware of the fact that many trials with a negative result
are not reported in the literature. Due to lack of space not all possible problems
in the execution of these trials are discussed. The reader is referred to other
volumes [3, 4].

Corticosteroids

The first studies were performed by Faupel [5] and Gobiet [6] in the late 1970s
(Table 1). Gobiet's study was in fact not a trial but a cohort study with historical
control. Faupel's study revealed a favorable dose-related effect. Their positive
results were not confirmed in subsequent trials in the United States, Nether-
lands and the United Kingdom [7 – 10]. Saul reported a positive effect in a specific group of so-called responders, but again this was not be confirmed in
other studies. A subsequent German multicenter study sponsored by Merck
looked at the effect of "ultrahigh" doses of a glucococorticoid. The result,
again, was disappointingly negative [11]. The Grumme study [12] reported a
positive result, but its design and analysis are controversial. In my opinion,
and in the view of EBIC and ABIC, routine administration of glucocorticoids
cannot be recommended in head-injured patients.

Reference	Effect on outcome	Effect on ICP
Faupel et al. 1976 [5]	+	
Cooper et al. 1979 [8]		–
Saul et al. 1981 [10]	–	
Braakman et al. 1983 [7]	–	
Dearden et al. 1986 [9]	–	–
Gaab et al. 1993 [11]	–	
Grumme et al. [12] 1995	(±)?	

Table 1. Effect of glucocorticoids

Barbiturates

The administration of high doses of barbiturates has a favorable effect on elevated ICP (Table 2). This is due to several distinct mechanisms. Lowering of
metabolic demands is one of them. Three randomized controlled trials have

Table 2. Barbiturates and ICP

Reference	Pentobarbital versus	Effect on ICP
Schwartz et al. 1984 [13]	Mannitol	−
Ward et al. 1985 [14]	Standard treatment	−
Eisenberg et al. 1988 [15]	Standard treatment	+

been performed [13–15]. None of these showed a favorable effect on outcome when barbiturates were compared with the administration of mannitol [13[, or standard treatment in a specific group of severely head-injured patients [14] or in the multicenter study by Eisenberg and coworkers [15] in cases of intractable ICP elevation. Administration of high-dose barbiturates may lower ICP and perhaps decrease mortality in a case of uncontrollable ICP, but its administration is not indicated as prophylactic management of ICP. The drug has important side effects, in particular serious hypotension. Further substudies such as those in patients with intact autoregulation are still necessary.

Dihydropyridines (Calcium Entry Blockers)

The large European multicenter trials HIT 1 and HIT 2 [16, 17] have shown that the routine administration of nimodipine in severe head injury has no positive effect on outcome. In a subgroup of HIT 2 a positive effect was seen in patients with subarachnoid hemorrhage on their initial CT. In the third trial, HIT 3 [18], including only patients who revealed a traumatic subarachnoid hemorrhage on their initial CT, a definite positive effect was identified, far more impressive than we had ever expected. In cases of traumatic subarachnoid hemorrhage the administration of nimodipine is, in my view, mandatory nowadays. Even the critical reviewers of the results of this trial in the *Journal of Neurosurgery* agreed on this.

Food

There are trials already performed and now underway which look at the value of administered certain foods or comparing enteral and parenteral food administration. Some of these are listed in Table 3 [18, 19].

Table 3. Nutrition and outcome

Reference	Result
Rapp et al. 1983 [20]	Early feeding reduces mortality
Hadley 1986 [23]	Parenteral and enteral same N-balance
Young 1987 [24]	More rapid recovery with better early nutrition; at 6 months no difference
Grahm 1989 [25]	Nasojejunal feeding gives better N-balance than gastric feeding

Anticonvulsants

Various trials have studied the effect of anticonvulsants on epilepsy. The overall result is that they reduce the incidence of early seizures but do not reduce that of late seizures [20, 21]

Mannitol

Trials on the effect of mannitol administration on ICP and other aspects of head injury management have been performed. Schwartz et al. [22] compared this to barbiturates and found it to be superior. Smith et al. [23] compared it to an empiric therapy and found the two to be of equal effect. Rather than discussing their results in detail, we consider here more recent trials that involve many European centers.

Currently there are two more types of drugs under investigation: the antioxidants PEG-SOD and Tirilazad. The American PEG-SOD trial had no positive result: the group receiving PEG-SOD did not show a statistically significant better outcome (not yet published). The results of the Tirilazad trials in Europe and the United States are reported in detail elsewhere in this book.

The other group of drugs under actual clinical investigation includes the NMDA antagonists, both competitive and noncompetitive. Three are examining the former [CGS 19755 (Selfotel) Ciba Geigy, EAA 494 (Saphir) Sandoz, Cerestat Boehringer-CNS] and the fourth is studying the latter (MK 801 Merck). There are also trials with other NMDA antagonists planned by other pharmaceutical companies. The Ciba trial with Selfotel has recently been stopped by their safety committee; details of their reasons are not yet available. The Sandoz trial, in collaboration with EBIC, admitted about 80 patients over the past 2 months, but requires over 800 patients. We can expect its result in 1998. The CNS Boehringer trial with Cerestat, also in collaboration with EBIC, starts soon. These drugs are very potent in animal experiments, but also have more important side effects than corticoids or nimodipine.

Conclusion

Of the drugs that have been tested in trials the only really effective one to date in patients with a traumatic subarachnoid hemorrhage has been nimodipine. Its effect seems so powerful that even in this small trial with a little over 100 patients significant results were obtained. This demonstrates once more that in the future trials should be performed in specific subgroups of head injury. The major remaining problem is to identify these groups in advance.

References

1. Anonymous (1984) Guidelines for initial management after head injury in adults. Suggestions from a group of neurosurgeons. BMJ 288: 983–985
2. Anonymous (1995) Guidelines for the management of severe head injury. A joint initiative of the American Association of Neurological Surgeons and The Brain Trauma Foundation. Brain Trauma Foundation
3. Pocock SJ (1987) Clinical trials. A practical approach. Wiley, Chichester
4. Spilker B (1991) Guide to clinical trials. Raven, New York
5. Faupel G, Reulen HJ, Muller D et al (1976) Double-blind study on the effects of steroids on severe closed head injury: In: Pappius HM, Feindel W (eds) Dynamics of brain edema. Springer, Berlin Heidelberg New York, pp 337–343
6. Gobiet, W Bock WJ, Liesgang J et al (1976) Treatment of acute cerebral edema with high dose of dexamethason: In: Beks JWF, Bosch DA, Brock M (eds) Intracranial pressure III. Springer, Berlin Heidelberg New York, pp 231–235
7. Braakman R, Schouten HJ, Blaauw-van Dishoeck M et al (1983) Megadose steroids in severe head injury. J Neurosurg 58: 326–330
8. Cooper PR, Moody S, Clark WK et al (1979) Dexamethasone and severe head injury. A prospective double-blind study. J Neurosurg 51: 307–316
9. Dearden NM, Gibson J, Mc Dowell DG et al (1986) Effect of high-dose dexamethasone on outcome from severe head injury. J Neurosurg 64: 81–88
10. Saul TG, Ducker TB, Salcman M et al (1981) Steroids in severe head injury. A prospective randomized clinical trial. J Neurosurg 54: 594–600
11. Gaab MR, Trost HA, Alcantara A et al (1994) "Ultrahigh" dexamethasone in acute brain injury. Results from a prospective randomized double-blind multicenter trial. Zentralbl Neurochir 55: 135–143
12. Grumme T, Baethmann A, Kolodziejczyk D (1995) Treatment of patients with severe head injury by triamcinolone: a prospective controlled multicenter trial of 396 cases. Res Exp Med 195: 217–229
13. Schwartz M, Tator C, Towed D et al (1984) The University of Toronto head injury treament study: a prospective randomized comparison of pentobarbital and mannitol. Can J Neurol Sci 11: 434–440
14. Ward JD, Becker DP, Miller JD et al (1985) Failure of prophylactic barbiturate coma treatment of severe head injury. J Neurosurg 62: 383–388
15. Eisenberg HM, Frankowski RF, Constant CF et al (1988) High-dose barbiturate control of elevated intracranial pressure in patients with severe head injury. J Neurosurg 69: 15–23
16. Bailey J, Bell A, Gray J et al (1991) A trial of the effect of nimodipine on outcome after head injury. Acta Neurochir 110: 97–105
17. European Study Group on Nimodipine in Severe Head Injury (1994) A multicenter trial on the efficacy of nimodipine on outcome after severe head injury. J Neurosurg 80: 797–804
18. Harders A, Kakarieka A, Braakman R et al (1996) Traumatic subarachnoid hemorrhage and its treatment with nimodipine. J Neurosurg 85: 82–89
19. Clifton GL, Robertson CS, Constant DF (1985) Enteral hyperalimentation in head injury. J Neurosurg 62: 186–193
20. Rapp RP, Young B, Twyman D et al (1983) The favorable effect of early parenteral feeding on survival in head injured patients. J Neurosurg 58: 906–912
21. Schwartz ML, Tator CH, Rowed DW (1984) The University of Toronto Head Injury treatment Study: a prospective randomized comparison of pento-barbital and mannitol. Can J Neurol Sci 11: 434–440
22. Smith HP, Kelly DL, Mc Wother JM et al (1986) Comparison of mannitol regimens in patients with severe head injury undergoing intracranial monitoring. J Neurosurg 65: 820–824
23. Hadley MN, Grahm TW, Harrington et al (1986) Nutritional support and neurotrauma: A critical review of early nutrition in forty-five acute head injury patients. Neurosurgery 19: 367–373
24. Young B, Ott L, Twyman D et al. (1987) The effect of nutritional support on outcome from severe head injury. J Neurosurg 67: 668–676
25. Grahm TW, Zadrozny DB, Harrington T (1989) Benefits of early jejunal hyperalimentation in the head-injured patient, Neurosurgery 25: 729–735

2 Pathophysiology of Brain Injury: An Overview

T.J. Kuhn

Introduction

During the last decade there was a decrease in mortality of severe brain injuries. In the same period the morbidity in brain-injured patients improved in our clinical experience. The publication on interactions between factors determining prognosis in populations of patients with severe head injury presented by Braakman [4] and the limits to classification and prognosis of severe head injury described by Frowein and coworkers [11] started with a large data bank on head-injured patients to observe prediction factors and prognosis. These studies led to better classifications of head injury and the limits set for clinically based prognosis and recovery. The Glasgow Coma Scale, introduced by Teasdale and Jennett in 1974, has become the 'gold standard' in the assessment of head injuries.

The improvement in outcome after brain injuries has become possible due to our better knowledge of the pathological, pathophysiological and biochemical changes following brain injury. Also better methods of monitoring during intensive care, such as intracranial pressure (ICP), brain tissue PO_2, cerebral perfusion pressure (CPP), and hemodynamic monitoring, and aggressive treatment may help to improve outcome following brain injuries. Early rehabilitation is also an important factor.

The history of research on the pathophysiology of brain injury started more than 200 years ago. It was the merit of the Scottish anatomist Alexander Monro in 1783 who hypothesized that "as substance of the brain, like that of the other solids of our body, is nearly incompressible, the quantity of blood within the head must be the same or nearly the same, at all times, whether in health or in disease, in life or after death." The studies from George Kellie, 1824, completed this hypothesis; Weed later set down the doctrine of 'Monro and Kellie' of the basic knowledge of pressure–volume conditions in the neurocranium. Cotugno reported in 1764 about the CSF-carrying spaces, the ventricular system, and the subarachnoid space. Magendie postulated in 1825 the circulation of CSF from the ventricular system to the subarachnoid space. Early experimental studies on ICP were performed by Cooper and Donders. Manometric measurements of ICP were conducted in the nineteenth century by Adamkiewicz [1] and others. This research contributed a lot of facts pertaining to the development of raised ICP after brain trauma. Emil von Bergmann described after first carrying out animal studies the "clinical signs of brain pressure" in respiratory, circulatory, and consciousness disturbances. Courtney postulated in 1899 [8] vasomotor paralysis after brain injury as a reason for circulatory arrest following increased ICP. Kocher's experiments on raised ICP inspired Harvey Cushing during his Europe visit in 1900 to perform his own investigations on brain pressure. In 1926 [7] Carter described the connection with raised pressure in CSF spaces and brain trauma and the better outcome after CSF drainage in brain-injured patients. In 1951 Guillaume and Janny were the first to perform continuous recording of intraventricular pressure in humans. These studies were further developed and published by Ryder and coworkers [28]. Later, Lundberg published his investigations about three distinct, well-defined ventricular fluid pressure fluctuations of different pattern magnitude and frequency [18,19]: A waves were recorded in situtations of moderately elevated ICP (patients complained of headache, nausea, and vomiting).

B waves are rhythmic oscillations with a frequency of 0.5 – 2/min (e. g., in conditions of periodic breathing such as Cheyne-Stokes syndrome, somnolence, or normal sleep) They are, as C waves, smaller, more rhythmic, and of limited clinical implications. Lundberg [18] also classified the severity of increased ICP:

- Severely increased: > 40 mm Hg
- Moderately increased: 20 – 40 mm Hg
- Slightly increased: 10 – 20 mm Hg

During the last 30 years our knowledge of the physiological and biochemical changes has developed increasingly, especially due to the research, for example of Miller [23 – 25], Marmorou and Tabbador [21], Rosner, Baethmann [3] and other scientists. There are still a lot of open questions in pathophysiological and biochemical problems following brain injury which require further investigation.

Axonal Damage

As a result of closed brain injury without radiological signs of primary brain damage on computed tomographic (CT) scan, diffuse axonal damage can develop. This axonal tissue damage, which is caused by deceleration – acceleration – trauma of the head, can only be diagnosed by histopathological examinations. Simultaneous development of damage on subcellular structures leads to neuroaxonal disturbances, which causes coma in the patient clinically.

Diffuse axonal injury (DAI), described by Adams and coworkers [2], causes prolonged coma in patients with brain injury, and is graded in three forms:

- Grade I: axonal damage in the white matter of the hemispheres, in the corpus callosum, cerebellum, and brainstem
- Grade II: focal damage in the corpus callosum
- Grade III: focal damage additionally in the rostral brainstem

Tissue damage in the brainstem causes a prolonged coma and is usually combined with focal leasons in the white matter. Investigations from Genarelli et al. [12] pointed out that the direction of an acceleration trauma has an important impact on the development of DAI. He reported that sagittal accelerations causes grade I DAI; lateral accelerations produce a high incidence of high grade DAI. Low-grade brain injuries can also be connected with DAI. For more information on this topic please refer to the chapter by Mennel, this volume.

Changes in Vascular Reactivity

Changes in vascular reaction and perfusion are a frequent consequence of brain injury. Changes in blood circulation have an unfavorable effect on cellular function and causes disturbances in biochemical and physiological processes in the ultrastructural metabolism of the cell. Changes in autoregulatory function of the brain vessels have been well described by Wei [37]. He performed the following types of experiments of dysfunction of brain vessels after brain trauma:

- Dilatation of arterioles immediately after trauma
- Decrease in vasoconstriction ability in hypocapnic conditions even in low-grade brain injuries
- Autoregulatoric vasodilatation in arterial hypotension is also possible in low-grade brain injuries
- In high-grade brain injuries vessels can lose their tonus, especially in arterial hypotension
- Reactive hyperemia in arterial hypoxic conditions is reduced in the injured brain

Changes in reactions of blood vessels are followed by changes in cerebral blood flow (CBF). In experimental conditions initial hyperemia is followed by a decrease in vessel resistance. This development can escalate up to a complete loss of autoregulatory function. Numerous further studies investigated the connection between autoregulatory dysfunction and outcome after brain injury. Different authors found both decrease and excessive increase of CBF; they did not find a dependence of changes in autoregulation to the grade and outcome after brain injury. Investigations in the early phase after injury (4–12 h), however, produced results in patients with a CBF on the infarction borderline of CBF of less than 16–18 ml/100 g per minute. Here a high mortality rate was found.

Ischemia After Severe Brain Injury

Graham and Adams [14] described in a postmortem study focal ischemic damage in brain sections after trauma in 80 % of cases. The distribution of these lesions was quite different. Ischemic lesions have been seen in particular in the cortex, hippocampus, basal ganglia, and the brainstem:

- Mass movement causes infra- or supratentorial herniation with compression of the feeding arteries
- Traction on feeding vessels causes ischemia or bleeding
- Vasospasm of the arteries can occur, i. e., in traumatic subarachnoid bleeding
- Increasing ICP and development of brain edema causes perfusion disturbances
- Autoregulatory functions of the brain vessels can be disturbed or destroyed
- Brain swelling can cause minimal perfusion, before ICP reaches high levels

The intracranial cerebral blood volume is fixed on CBF within the limits of cerebral autoregulation of 50–150 mm Hg. The CBF is modulated by metabolic, chemical, and neurogenic factors and is independent of the calculated parameter CPP.

The borderline for ischemic endangered perfusion of brain tissue is a flow rate of less than 16–18 ml/100 mg per minute. Siesjö [30] reported about disturbances in neurogenic activity of neurons when the CBF rate is reduced to less than 12 ml/100 mg per minute. In this situation the homeostasis of the cell is disturbed; the result is a potassium efflux and a calcium influx through the cell membrane. The cell membrane is consequently destroyed and the membrane functions such as sodium/potassium pump are lost [30].

Postmortem angiographic investigations described a significant correlation between trauma-induced vasospasm and following ischemia with tissue destruction. On this topic current investigations are searching for an answer to the question of whether calcium antagnoists are a useful tool to prevent tSAB-induced vasospasm as a cerebroprotective measure in brain trauma with accompanying traumatic subarachnoid hemorrhage. The vasospasm itself causes reduction of CBF and is disposed to the following pathophysiological steps to ischemic lesions.

Tissue Damage Following Ischemia–Reperfusion Damage

Vasomotor paralysis following damage of the brainstem and its vascular supply can be caused by brain trauma. In the postparalysis period an increase of CBF occurs. This causes increased brain swelling and at least an increase in ICP.

Iatrogenic procedures, such as operative decompressive craniotomy in therapy-resistant brain pressure elevation, can be followed by vasomotor paralysis. Consequently, the initial increase in blood flow will be followed by an increase in ICP. Due to the raised ICP minimal perfusion with the risk of hypoxia and ischemia and tissue damage will occur.

Brain Edema

Traumatic brain edema, either primary or secondary, is a central pathophysio-logical and pathobiochemical problem following brain injury. Apart from problems in the development of the actual cellular damage, the difficulties are well known in therapy of brain edema and raised ICP.

Go et al. [13] described the primary vasogenic development of brain edema in the early period after trauma. Cellular swelling is due to inadequate func-tion of the sodium/potassium pump with an increase in sodium influx into the cell, followed by fluid shift. A potassium efflux into the extracellular space can also be noticed. Following this shift of electrolytes and water, the organization and subcellular function of the organelles becomes disturbed. If the sodium/potassium pump is defective, the membrane function declines and, finally, the cell structure is completely destroyed. The potassium efflux into the extracel-lular space can be measured immediately after the trauma. The potassium eff-lux liberates neurotransmitters, such as excitatory amino acids (EAA) and glu-tamate. The liberation of glutamate induces further potassium efflux and cal-cium influx into intact cellular structures. This excessive intracellular calcium level activates proteases. The biological activity of these proteases causes the collapse of the cellular membrane and its connections to other cells and the destruction of the plasma membrane.

Activation of phospholipase C following brain injuries has to be expected. This enzyme liberates arachidonic acid. The enzyme cyclooxygenase converts arachidonic acid to the endoperoxid prostaglandine G2 (PGG2). Prostaglan-din-hyperoxidase converts prostaglandin G2 to prostaglandin H2; this enzyme causes the formation of free oxygen radicals (O_2^-) in the presence of NADH or NADPH. These biochemical interactions start in the walls of the blood vessels immediately after the brain trauma.

Investigations by Ikeda and Long [16] and Povlishock [27] demonstrated that free oygen radicals and hydrogen peroxide (H_2O_2) in the presence of mole-cular iron react to the highly toxic radical OH^-. This free radical can interact with nearly all molecules which are present in the living cell.

Mediators of vascular and parenchymal mechanisms in secondary brain damage are different. Investigations from Baethmann et al. [3] and Unterberg et al. [31–33] described the role of bradykinin, arachidonic acid, histamine, leukotrienes, serotonin, and free radicals in the pathogenesis of vasogenic brain edema. Vasogenic brain edema is one important factor in the develop-ment of secondary brain tissue damage.

Bradykinin can induce brain edema by increasing blood–brain barrier per-meability and enhancing blood pressure due to arterial dilatation and venous constriction. After experimental trauma there is an increase in bradykinin concentration in brain tissue. Arachidonic acid also opens the blood–brain barrier for large tracers. There are no vasoactive effetcts. The edema is associ-ated with an increase in levels of arachidonic acid in brain tissue. This media-tor is also able to induce cytotoxic edema. Histamine's function has been described in vasoactive functions, i. e., dilatation of brain vessels. In contrast to histamine, leukotriene leads to vasoconstriction of cerebral arteries but not to extravasation of fluids.

Free oxygen radicals are pathobiochemically able to cause an increase in CBF following vasodilatation of blood vessels. This process raises the ICP by increasing the intracranial blood volume. This is an important reason for vasogenic brain edema development.

Free oxygen radicals can also induce mechanisms for the development of the cytotoxic brain edema:

- Lipid peroxidation
- Emptying of calcium stores
- Impeding of enzyme functions
- Destroying of mitochondrium
- Damaging of DNA
- Damaging of cellular membranes

Clinical trials on treatment with free oxygen radical scavengers (polyethylene glycol-conjugated superoxide dismutase) have been conducted. Muizelaar et al. [26] published the results of the phase II trial and summarized that there are still problems in treatment with lazaroids in daily practice. Further investigations and results can be expected. The preliminary results of these trials are published in the guidelines of treatment of severe head injuries in Chap. 7, this volume.

Bullock et al [6] reported about clinical investigations to determine the incidence and time course of abnormalities in the blood–brain barrier after both cerebral contusion and acute subdural hematoma and established the relationship between CBF and abnormalities of the blood–brain barrier and the extent of edema, demonstrated by T2-weighted magnetic resonance imaging (MRI). These studies showed that edema, shown by MRI and CT scanning, is a universal finding even early after contusion and that a focal zone of low CBF in relation to the contusions was always present. A defect of blood–brain barrier was established by pertechnetate-SPECT investigations and demonstrated that, particularly early after injury, contusion edema is predominantly cytotoxic in nature.

Intracranial Pressure

One of the most important pathophysiological signs of brain injury is the development of raised ICP. An increase in ICP does not occur as long as compensatory mechanisms are able to divert CSF from the intracranial to the intraspinal subarachnoid compartment. Another mechanism of compensation is the reduction of cerebral blood volume (CBV) by cerebral vasoconstriction.

One reason for raised ICP is the brain edema, which can be caused by different pathological processes, such as brain trauma, brain tumor, or mass bleeding. Closed severe brain injuries are often associated with brain edema caused by the above described pathophysiological genesis of vasogenic or cytotoxic edema or by traumatic mass lesions.

Other reasons for raised ICP are primary traumatic intracranial mass lesions, such as epidural, subdural, or intracerebral hematomas, hydrocephalus and brain tumors with midline shifting.

Genarelli et al. [12] introduced two types of intracranial hypertension following experimental head injury in primates: brain swelling, which occurs during a short time by vasodilatation, and congestion of the traumatized brain area (focal edema). This type was also described by Bruce et al. [5] as a main reason for raised ICP in children after brain trauma. The other type is a diffuse swelling of both hemispheres (generalized or malignant edema). This type occurs 2–3 days after injury, especially in younger patients. The compensatory spaces are compressed and the ventricular system and the basal cisterns are absent at CT examination. Genarelli suggested that this type of brain swelling is an effect of blood–brain barrier following cerebral vasodilatation.

There are two types of brain edema, which have to be distinguished:

1. Vasogenic edema
2. Cellular-cytotoxic edema.

Vasogenic edema is caused by a breakdown in the blood–brain barrier and increased permeability of capillaries with extravasation of fluid into the extravascular, i. e., interstitial, space. This type is mostly combined with severe brain injuries. The fluid shift to the extracellular spaces causes an osmotic gradient from intra- to extracellular spaces and causes a vicious circle.

Cellular edema is the result of brain swelling and dysfunction of cellular membranes and later cellular organelles. The electrolyte equilibrium is disturbed by dysfunction of adenosine-triphosphatase (ATPase). Later, cell dysfunction and cell destruction occur.

Findings from Monro and Kellie in the eighteenth and nineteenth century described the character of intracranial components, brain tissue mass, blood vessels, blood volume, and CSF in the intra-and extracerebral spaces. The so-called doctrine of Monro and Kellie postulates that changes in the volume of one of the three compartments is only possible by reciprocal changes in the volume of the other compartments.

Measured on different points in the cerebrum, ICP can present with various values. ICP in the supratentorial area may be different from ICP in the spinal subarachnoid space. Increasing supratentorial ICP can be observed with ICP decreasing in the infratentorial space.

The normal value of ICP in adults is defined as 0–15 mm Hg. The ICP is modulated slowly by respiratory und quickly by cardiac effects. The physiological steady state of ICP is mathematically defined by the equation:

$$ICP = I_f \times R_o + P_v$$

where I_f = CSF production, R_o = CSF drain resistance, P_v = central venous pressure).

The production of CSF is constant in a large distance of ICP. There is a decrease in CSF production during high ICP levels.

From this point of view the pressure – volume relation was defined. First, in the compensated phase of increasing volume, the increase in pressure is small. In the next step, the ICP rises exponentially and at the least the pressure rises very steeply.

The volume/pressure elastance is defined by the pressure change following the volume changes:

$$E = dP/dV$$

The slope of the curve is determined by the elasticity of the brain to volume changes, usually referred to as compliance:

$$C = dV/dP$$

Different pathological factors have an effect on the level of ICP. The development of the pressure – volume curve does not follow linear conditions (Fig. 1). The curve is influenced by the different pathophysiological factors elastance, compliance, blood flow und venous drainage, as summarized below:

- The volume of a mass lesion
- Changes in absorption of CSF
- Changes in CSF volume
- Compliance of brain tissue
- Cerebrovascular volume and blood pressure
- Venous drainage of the brain

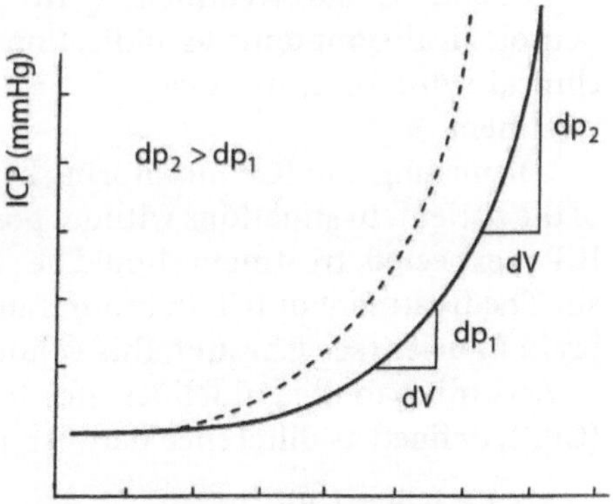

Fig. 1. Intracranial pressure volume relation. Volume (ml): low increase of ICP (dp_1) after increase of volume (dV) by normal compliance. Extensive increase of ICP (dp_2) with the same increase of volume (dV) in a situation with decreased compliance: progressive increase of ICP

The development of untreated raised ICP is limited in cases of herniation of the brain to anatomically preformed locations, i. e., infra- or supratentorially. Herniation is stressed by mass movements or the summation effects of mass movement and brain edema development. During this herniation process different focal neurologic, i. e., clinical signs, can occur:

- Midbrain disturbances and brainstem ischemia with the clinical signs of unconsciousness, circulatory and cardiac disturbances, dyspnea and dysfunction of the descending systems, diabetes insipidus
- Termination of CSF flow and ICP increase based on hydrocephalus
- Compression of n. III with mydriasis of one or both pupils
- Compression of the medulla oblongata with extension or flexion synergisms and or respiratory disturbances or respiratory arrest

ICP Monitoring and Treatment

The monitoring of ICP can be measured at different locations of the brain and with different techniques. One location is the lateral ventricle, where fluid drainage and ICP = IVP monitoring is possible. Other locations are the epidural space above the hemispheres (epidural measurement) or the white matter (intraparenchymal measurement).

Measured at different places of the CNS, ICP can present with various values. ICP in the supratentorial area may be different to the pressure into the subarachnoid space. Increasing ICP supratentorially can be observed. A decrease in ICP can be measured in the infratentorial space.

The normal value of ICP in adults is defined from 0–15 mm Hg. Raised ICP has to be expected in nearly all situations of severe brain injury and other pathological processes into the neurocranium. Intracranial hypertension is an emergency situation and has to be monitored and treated aggressively as soon as possible after trauma to prevent cell dysfunction, circulatory disturbances, and secondary ischemic tissue damage. Some authorities recommend treating raised ICP from levels greater than 15 mm Hg.

The authors start treatment up from levels of 20 mm Hg. In many situations neurological symptoms as indication for raised ICP cannot be noticed. The clinical symptoms are unspecific. So early exact diagnosis is necessary for treatment.

CT imaging and ICP monitoring has to be performed early after admission of the patient. In situations without possibilities for diagnosis but where raised ICP is expected, treatment should be started even without an accurate diagnosis. The treatment of ICP in brain trauma is based on the guidelines in severe brain injuries (see Chesnut, this volume).

According to the guidelines the monitoring of cerebral perfusion pressure (CPP), defined as difference between middle arterial blood pressure and ICP

$$MABP\text{-}ICP = CPP$$

has become of great importance in monitoring and treatment of elevated ICP. This parameter, which is correlated with oxygen partial pressure in brain tissue, can be focussed on therapy of hemodynamics. This parameter can be monitored very easily without any instruments. The value should be more than 60 mm Hg. It is of great importance in connection with the other neuromonitoring parameters ICP, $P(ti)O_2$ and MABP.

Continuous Monitoring of Brain Tissue Oxygenation

A new monitoring method is the examination of the oxygen partial pressure in brain tissue. This method became possible with the development of the LICOX PO_2 probe. This PO_2 probe is a Clark-type probe, developed for this investigation in humans by Fleckenstein and coworkers (Kiel, FRG). It is an invasive method; the probe can be implanted into the white matter through a mini-burr hole. Another possibility is monitoring of oxygen partial pressure in CSF, measured in the ventricular system.

Oxygen ions can diffuse through a semipermeable diaphragm and generate an electric current. The current intensity is registered and transformed into the tissue oxygen partial pressure by the LICOX device. Investigations by Flekkenstein, Maas [20], Meixensberger [22], Unterberg and the authors [17] established the "normal values" of this new parameter. They found a correlation between $P(ti)O_2$ and cerebral perfusion pressure and also to the middle arterial blood pressure. Some therapy-related events upon increasing $P(ti)O_2$ values have been described, such as during changes in hyperventilation, barbiturate therapy, and treatment with osmodiuretics. This new parameter will become more importance to assess the danger of hypoxia during elevated ICP in order to prevent secondary ischemic brain damage. A detailed assessment of this method is well described in Chap. 12 by J. Meixensberger, this volume, and Chap. 13 by A. Unterberg.

Principles of Treatment of Raised ICP

A joint venture of the Brain Trauma Foundation, the American Association of Neurological Surgens, and the Joint Section on Neurotrauma and Critical Care published the Guidelines for the Management of Severe Head Injury. Based on this therapeutic guideline the following maneuvers have to be applied during the treatment of intracranial hypertension.

In severely head-injured patients episodes of arterial hypotension and hypoxia have to be avoided. The systolic blood pressure should be kept above 90 mm Hg and the PaO_2 < 60 mm Hg by arterial blood gas analysis must be rapidly corrected to improve outcome. A CPP > 70 mm Hg should also be maintained.

Comatose head-injured patients (GOS 3-8) with an abnormal CT scan should undergo ICP monitoring in the ICU. Comatose patients with normal CT scan should only undergo monitoring when two of the following criteria are fullfilled at the time of admission: age over 40 years, unilateral or bilateral motor posturing, or systolic blood pressure under 90 mm Hg.

The treatment of elevated ICP should be initiated at an upper threshold of 20-25 mm Hg In temporal lobe lesions treatment should begin at a threshold of 15 mm Hg.

Prophylactic hyperventilation of severely head-injured patients should be strictly avoided in order to prevent a reduction of CBF. CBF reduction does not reduce ICP and may cause a loss of autoregulation. The outcome of brain-injured patients treated with prophylactic hyperventilation is worse.

The bolus administration of mannitol is recommended according to the Guidelines for the reduction of ICP. Serum osmolalities should be kept below 320 mOsm/l.

Elevated ICP refractory to conventional treatment is a subject of high-dose barbiturate therapy. The prophylactic use of barbiturates is not indicated. Barbiturates should only be used in ICU with appropriate monitoring devices.

The use of glycocorticoids in the treatment of severe head injury is due to all available evidence not useful. They do not reduce ICP or improve outcome.

Full nutritional support is to be applied by the seventh day after head injury, either enteral or parenteral, containing at least 15 % of calories as protein.

The majority of studies do not support the use of antiseizure prophylaxis in head injury for the onset of late postraumatic seizures.

Summary

Brain injury results in local and/or diffuse neural damage. Primary and secondary brain damage has to be distinguished. Primary brain damage is caused by a trauma and presents in mass lesion defects. Secondary brain damage follows a trauma presenting dysfunction of vascular autoregulation, hypoxia, hypoxemia (anemic, respiratory, and circulatory), ischemia and at least tissue damage.

The knowledge of basic underlying concepts of the pathophysiology following brain injury leads to a better understanding of the problems in brain injury and the specific therapeutic strategies.

References

1. Adamkiewicz A (1890) Über das Wesen des vermeintlichen Hirndrucks und die Princi-pien der Behandlung der sogenannten Hirndrucksymptome. Sitzungsberichte d. kais. Akademie d. Wissenschaften, Bd. XCIX, Abtlg. III, Vienna, November, 1890
2. Adams JH, Doyle D, Ford I, Genarelli TA, Graham DI, McLellan DR (1989) Diffuse axonal injury in head injury: definition, diagnosis and grading. Histopathology 15: 49–59
3. Baethmann, A, Oettinger W, Rothenfußer W, Kempski O, Unterberg A, Geiger R (1980) Brain edema factors: current state with particular reference to plasma constituents and gluatamate. Adv Neurol 28 171–195
4. Braakman R (1978) Interactions between factors determining prognosis in poupulations of patients with severe head injury. Adv Neurosurg 5: 12-15
5. Bruce DA, Alavi A, Bilaniuk L et al (1981) Diffuse cerebral swelling following head injuries in children: the syndrome of malignant brain edema. J Neurosurg 138: 271–273
6. Bullock R, Statham P, Patterson D, Wyper D, Hadley D, Teasdale E (1990) The time course of vasogenic oedema atfer focal human head injury – evidence from SPECT mapping of blood brain barrier defects. Acta Neurochir Suppl (Wien) 51: 286–288
7. Carter BN (1926) Diagnosis and treatment of fractures of the skull as developed in the Cincinnati General Hospital. Ann Surg 83: 182–195

8. Courtney JW, Traumatic cerebral edema: its pathology and surgical treatment – a critical study.
9. Cushing H (1901) Concerning a definite regulatory mechanisms of the vaso-motor center which controls blood pressure during cerebral compression. Johns Hopkins Hosp Bull 12: 290–292
10. Cushing H (1903) Some experimental and clinical observations concerning states of increased intracranial pressure. Am J Med Sci 124: 375–400
11. Frowein RA, Steinmann HW, Auf der Haar K, Terhaag D, Karimi-Nejad A (1978) Limits to classification and prognosis of severe head injury. Adv Neurosurg 5: 16
12. Genarelli TA, Thibault LE, Adams JH, Graham DI, Thompson CJ, Marcincin, RP (1985) Diffuse axonal injury and traumatic coma of the central nervous system., Raven, New York, pp 169–193
13. Go KG (1991) The blood–brain and blood–cerebrospinal fluid barriers. In: Go KG (ed) Cerebral pathophysiology. An integral approach with some emphasis on clinical implications. Elsevier, Amsterdam, pp 1–65
14. Graham DI, Adams JH (1971) Ischemic brain damage in fatal head injuries. Lancet 1: 365–266
15. Guidelines on severe brain injury (1996). J Neurotrauma (Suppl) 12
16. Ikeda Y, Long DM (1990) The molecular basis of brain injury and brain edema: the role of oxygen free radicals. J Neurosurg 27: 1–11
17. Kuhn TJ, Bauer BL (1996) Multimodal neuromonitoring based on CPP and $P(ti)O_2$ in patients with severe brain injury. In: International Proceedings of the Division of Intensive Care Medicine, 1996. Monduzzi, Bologna, pp 687–691
18. Lundberg N (1960) Continuous recording and control of ventricular fluid pressure in neurosurgical practice. Acta Psychiatr Neurol Scand 36 (Suppl 149): 1–193
19. Lundberg N, Kjallquist A, Bien C (1959) Reduction of increased intracrnial pressure by hyperventilation. Acta Psychiatr Neurol Scand 34 (Suppl 139): 4–64
20. Maas AIR, Fleckenstein W, Jong de DA, Santbrink van H (1993) Monitoring cerebral oxygenation: experimental studies and preliminary results of the continuous monitoring of cerebrospinal fluid and brain tissue oxygen tension. Acta Neurochir Suppl (Wien) 59: 50–57
21. Marmarou A, Tabbador K (1987) Intracranial pressure: physiology and pathophysiology. In: Cooper PR (ed) Head injury. Williams and Wilkins, Baltimore, pp 159–176
22. Meixensberger J, Dings J, Roosen K (1993) Studies of tissue PO2 in normal and pathological human brain cortex. Acta Neurochir Suppl (Wien) 59: 58–63
23. Miller JD, Stanek A, Langfitt TW (1972) Concepts of cerebral perfusion pressure and vascular compression during intracranial hypertension. Prog Brain Res 35: 411–432
24. Miller JD, Becker DP, Ward JD et al (1977) Significance of intracranial hypertension in severe head injury. J Neurosurg 47: 503–516
25. Miller JD, Becker DP, Ward JD, Sullivan HG, Adams WE, Rosser MJ (1977) Significance of intracranial hypertension in severe head injury. J Neurosurg 47: 503–516
26. Muizelaar JP, Marmarou A, Young HF, Choi SC, Wolf A, Schneider RI, Kontos HA (1993) Improving the outcome of severe head injury with the oxygen radical scavenger polyethylene glycol-conjugated superoxide dsimutase: a phase II trial. J Neurosurg 78: 375–382
27. Povlishock TJ (1992) Traumatically induced axonal injury: pathogenesis and pathobiological implications. Brain Pathol 2: 1–12
27a. Rosner MJ, Becker DP (1987) Origin and evolution of plateau waves. J Neurosurgery 21: 147–155
28. Ryder HW, Espey FF, Kimpbell FD (1952) The mechanism of the change in cerebrospinal fluid pressure following an induced change int the volume of the fluid space. J Lab Clin Med 41: 428–435
29. Shalmon E, Caron, MJ, Becker DP (1996) Intracranial pressure: pathology and pathophysiology. In: Tindall GT, Cooper PR, Barrow DL (eds) The practice of neurosurgery, vol 1. Williams and Wilkins, Baltimore
30. Siesjö BK (1992) Pathophysiology and tratment of focal cerebral ischemia, part I. Pathophysiology. J Neurosurg 77: 169–194
31. Unterberg A, Wahl M, Hammersen F, Baethman A (1987a) Permeability and vasomotor response of cerebral vessels during exposure to arachidonic acid. Acta Neuropathol 73: 209–219

32. Unterberg A, Wahl M, Baethmann A (1988) Effects of free radicals on permeability and vasomotor response of cerebral vessels. Acta Neuropathol 76: 238–244
33. Unterberg A, Polk T, Ellis E, Marmarou A (1990)Enhancement of infusion induced brain edema by mediator compounds. Adv Neurol 52: 355–358
34. Wahl M, Kuschinsky W (1984) The dilating effect of histamine on pial arteries of cats and ist mediation by H2-mediators. Circ Res 44: 161–165
35. Wahl M, Unterberg A, Whalley ET, Baethmann A, Young AR Edvinsson L, Wagner FFW (1986a)Cerebrovascular effects of bradykinin. In: Owman C, Hardebo JE (eds) Neural regulation of brain circulation. Elsevier, New York, pp 419–430
36. Wedd LH, McKibben PS (1919) Pressure changes in cerebrospinal fluid following intravenous injections of soultions of various concentrations. Am J Physiol 48: 512–530
37. Wei EP, Dietrich WD, Povlishock TJ, Navari RM, Kontos HA (1980) Functional, morphological and metabolic abnormalities of the cerebral microcirculation after concussive brain injuries in cats. CircRes 46: 37–47

3 The Morphology of Traumatic Head Injury

H.D. Mennel

Introduction

Traumatic head and brain injuries affect nervous tissue, in which regeneration is possible only to a very limited extent. Restitution of function seems to be the crucial problem in all kinds of nervous system damage. Thus the concept of neuroprotection has been developed for both endogeneous degenerative and traumatic conditions in the nervous system [4]. However, to date positive results from neuroprotective intervention have been obtained only in experimental settings. Neuroprotection is a preventive means, aimed at minimizing the brain injuries sequelae that are due to secondary changes such as edema or circulatory disturbances [7]. Brain injury and primary ischemic damage are both pathological conditions in which the sequence of secondary changes may impair the patient more than the original blow.

Traditionally, open and closed head injury are dealt with separately, since the danger of secondary infection is minimal in the latter. Furthermore, the analysis of open head injury nowadays is the domain of forensic pathology, stemming historically from wartime pathology. However, the morphology of the damaged tissue in open and closed head injuries is basically the same. We therefore deal with open head injury only briefly.

In closed head injury there is often a considerable discrepancy between the clinical status, on one hand, and the extent of tissue damage, on the other. This is especially true for "commotio cerebri," a brain concussion defined by Spatz [17] as "traceless" within the nervous matter itself, despite the severe clinical status of the patient. This discrepancy can also be seen in "contusio cerebri," a brain contusion in which the severe clinical condition of the patient may be combined with only small contusional lesions. Spatz coined the term Rindenprellungsherde, meaning literally cortical contusional foci, as the main pathological counterpart of substantial brain injury. In such conditions it may be feasible to distinguish between the primary event and the cascade of subsequent processes. The latter may provide a target for the mentioned neuroprotective efforts.

More recently, however, a primary condition has been described, primarily in English-language reports, which has been termed "diffuse axonal injury (DAI). This type of damage is thought to originate as a whole at the very time of the blunt head injury. If this is true, the opportunity for neuroprotection would be considerably reduced. The first observations of the pathological changes associated with this condition were made by Strich in 1956 [18].

Although the concept of diffuse axonal injury is now firmly established, several diffuse forms of brain trauma are distinguished today. DAI represents the most important subgroup and is regarded as primary diffuse brain injury. Diffuse secondary brain injury – a concept introduced by Symonds [20, 21] – is considered to comprise the late sequelae of contusional lesions, thus explaining the discrepancy between early and late clinical phenomena; ongoing mental, behavioral and neurological deficits and disabilities in contrast to the immediate loss of consciousness, that can be completely reversible.

Adams [1] has described the four following subtypes of diffuse traumatic brain injury: (a) diffuse axonal brain injury, (b) hypoxic brain damage, (c) brain edema, and (d) diffuse vascular damage. Only the diffuse axonal injury should be considered as a primary event.

A possible final consequence of a localized traumatic focus (e. g., extracerebral or even intracerebral traumatic hemorrhage or deep lacerations) is mass displacement. This mass displacement has also been called traumatic "compressio cerebri." Traditionally the term "compressio cerebri" is applied equally to two common types of early or late traumatic sequelae, namely epidural and subdural hemorrhage. These are both of considerable clinical significance and even today sometimes pose diagnostic problems. The advent of imaging methods, however, has greatly facilitated the diagnostic and therapeutic handling of these conditions.

This presentation discusses the pathological features of each of the traumatic conditions and their sequelae, closing with a comment on the different concepts.

Closed Head Injury

Diffuse Axonal Injury

This condition may be regarded in either a narrow or a broad sense. The narrow notion of the concept holds that DAI consists primarily of microscopic damage to the white matter. However, DAI can be divided into the following three components, two of which are visible macroscopically, while the third can be verified only by histological examination: (a) a focal, often small hemorrhage in the corpus callosum, (b) focal damage in the dorsolateral (part of the) upper brain stem, and (c) diffuse injury to the axons. If the two former abnormalities are both present, it is resonable to infer the presence of diffuse axonal injury. However, confirmation of the diagnosis of DAI depends upon the microscopic examination of the axons within the white matter. Thus, if the macroscopically visible components are absent, it is easy to miss the diagnosis of this condition. Likewise in severe brain injury with multiple foci of damage, including the corpus callosum and dorsolateral upper brainstem the presence of diffuse axonal injury may be overlooked. Advocates of this type of injury suggest that DAI may have a higher incidence than thought, owing to current underdiagnosis.

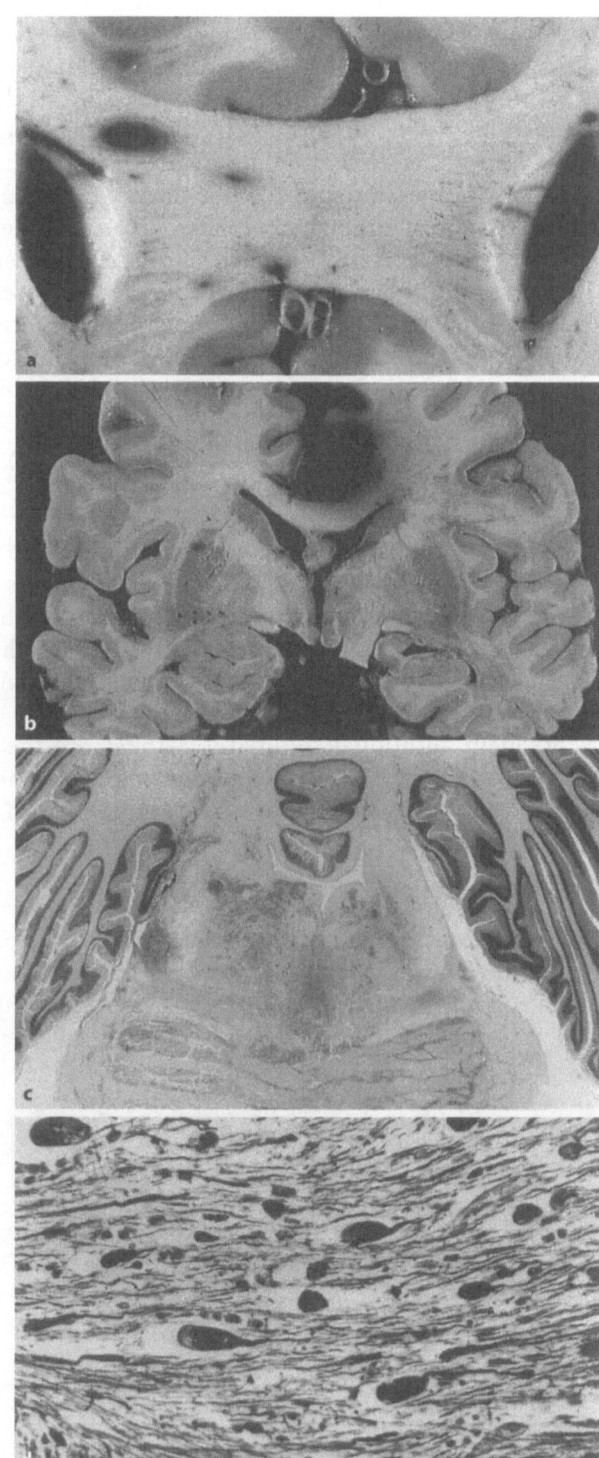

Fig. 1a–d. Morphology of diffuse axonal injury and related conditions. **a** Small hemorrhage in the rostal corpus callosum. This hemorrhage presents as oval bleeding in the lateral part of the rostrum corporis callosi. Note two other bleeding points on the opposite side and next to the midline. **b** Larger hemorrhage next to the cerebral midline, so called "gliding contusion." **c** Histology of the brainstem component of diffuse axonal injury. Note unilateral dorsal hemorrhage. Cresyl-violet staining. **d** Retraction bulbs of axons, impregnated by silver method. From [1]

The pathological change seen within the corpus callosum during the early stages of traumatic injury one or more small hemorrhages between the white fibers (Fig. 1a) adjacent to or reaching over the midline. Later, when shrinkage of the callosal structure occurs, the hemorrhage organizes, and we find one or more cysts or softenings. White fibers and axons are replaced by glial fibers, and siderophages, indicative of the former bleed, are found.

The changes within the dorsolateral region of the midbrain are very similar in nature. They present as small uni- or bilateral bleeds that very often involve the upper cerebellar peduncle (Fig. 1c). They are liquefied and eventually become small cystic necroses. Finding these conditions together is considered a very strong indication for the presence of the third component, i. e., the axonal damage, which, however, must always be verified by special histological methods.

In patients surviving this kind of injury for only a few days one can detect eosinophilic and/or argyrophilic "retraction balls" (Fig. 1d), indicating nonspecific alterations in damaged axons, originally described and named by Cajal et al. in 1959 [6]. These are found in the white matter of the cerebral and cerebellar hemispheres. After a few weeks clusters of microglial cells can be demonstrated within the injured white matter; within a few months wallerian degeneration of the long tracts occurs. Finally, the white matter is slightly diminished, the ventricles are mildly enlarged, and the corpus callosum is shrunken.

Frequent additional traumatic changes are the so-called "gliding contusions"; small hemorrhages next to the midline in the neighborhood of the falx cerebri (Fig. 1b) or in the area of the ammons horn [3].

Traumatic Contusional Foci

Traumatic contusional foci (traumatischer Rindenprellungsherd) are traditionally thought to occur as the most frequent feature of closed head injury. The predilection sites are the frontobasal and frontotemporal regions. A traumatic

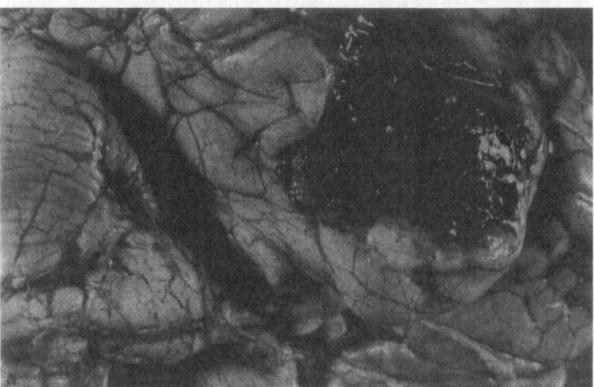

Fig. 2a – d. Cerebral cortical contusion. **a** Fresh cortical contusion on the lateral aspect of the temporal lobe presents as circumscript hemorrhage covering the contusional foci.

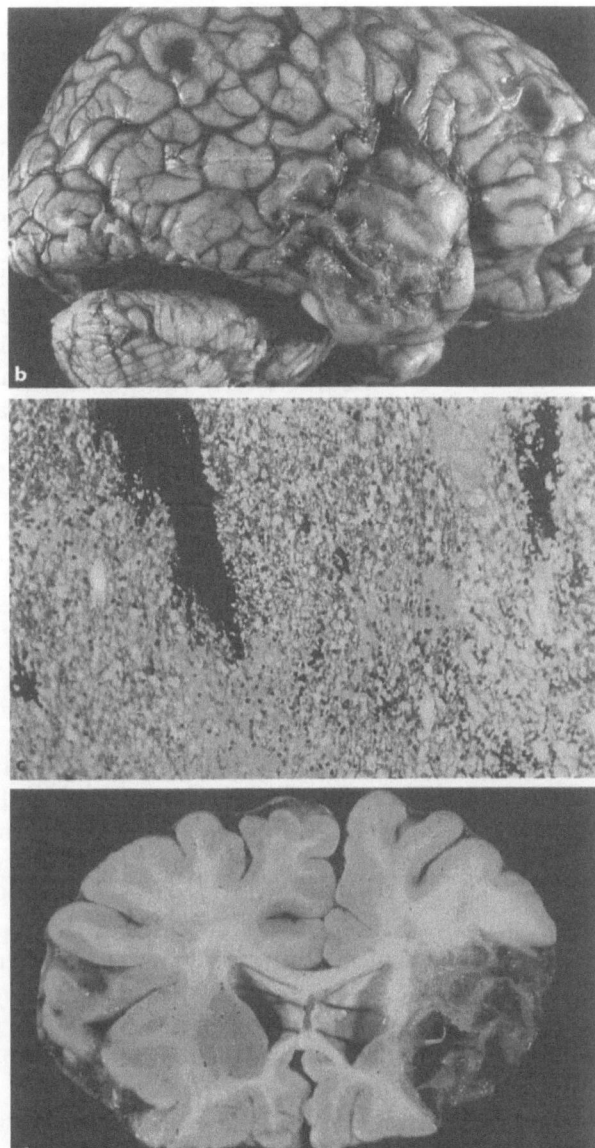

Fig. 2b Final stage of (different?) cortical contusions in the frontal, parietal, and temporal regions. The center of the cortical convolutions are affected resulting in the formation of schizogyria.
c Fresh contusional focus in the histological preparation. Note direct focal small bleeds. Diffuse edema and necrotic changes in cells. Trichrom, × 250.
d End-stage of localized traumatic injury comprising more than one cortical convolution. This is the French état vermolu. Note asymmetry of inner ventricular system

contusional focus always lies on the uppermost part of a cortical convolution and is considered to be the consequence of an acceleration motion. In its early stage it appears as a wedge-shaped hemorrhagic necrosis (Fig. 2a,c). Since it is situated in the immediate neighborhood of the subarachnoid space, a mild subarachnoidal hemorrhage is usually found, as confirmed by spinal fluid analysis. Even after weeks or months this fluid contains siderophages, which can be demonstrated in cytological preparations.

The necrosis is progressively organized by resorption of the necrotic material through fat granule cells. The final stage presents as a triangular indentation on the upper surface of a convolution, termed "schizogyria" (Fig. 2b).

Focal cortical contusions may occur at the site of the action of the force itself (coup focus) or in the opposite cortical region (contrecoup damage). The frequency with which either coup or contrecoup foci develop depends upon the direction and mechanism of the accelerating force. Thus an injury that hits the skull from the occipital to frontal direction almost exclusively yields fronto- and temporobasal traumatic foci. The distribution, however, is not the same if the force acts from the lateral or frontal direction.

The characteristic shape, localization, and distribution of contusional necroses has produced various theories as to the mechanism of their pathogenesis [14]. The most astonishing finding was the formation of contrecoup foci in over 95 % of cases, when the blow occurs at the occipital region. If the head is injured by a laterally acting force, the contusional foci are found in the coup and contrecoup position in almost equal numbers. If contusions affect more than one convolution, and the arachnoid is ruptured, in Europe this is known as "laceration" (Fig. 3a) [24]. The contusions are transformed into multiple scars on the convolutional surface [16]. Their impressive shape is expressed by the very descriptive French term état vermolu (Fig. 2d).

Traumatic Intracerebral Hemorrhage

Traumatic intracerebral hemorrhage occurs less frequently than traumatic contusional cortical foci but represents one of the more common consequences of head injury. It may present as either small or large white matter mass hemorrhage, designated "atypical" from both the clinical and pathological point of view. This must be differentiated from typical mass hemorrage, which usually originates as a consequence of long-standing elevated blood pressure. Hypertonic bleeding most commonly affects central structures such as the capsula interna or putamen-claustrum region, thalamus, brainstem or cerebellum. In contrast, traumatic hemorrhage is preferentially localized to the more peripherally situated lobi of the brain, therefore thus qualifying as atypical from the pathological viewpoint (Fig. 3b). Although lobar bleeds in general have various pathogenic causes, an important and not rare cause is closed head injury [13].

Traumatic bleeds within the brain parenchyma may be the cause of mass displacement, especially when combined with collateral edema. Life-threatening herniations beneath the falx cerebri and tentorial notches, and mass displacement through the foramen magnum may result [26]. The cascade of events leading to downward herniation is accompanied by characteristic clinical signs at each step. Due to the impact of imaging methods in neurological sciences, the course of events during mass displacement has become common knowledge in diagnostic routine. Formerly, neuropathology and forensic pathology dealt with these conditions [10, 11].

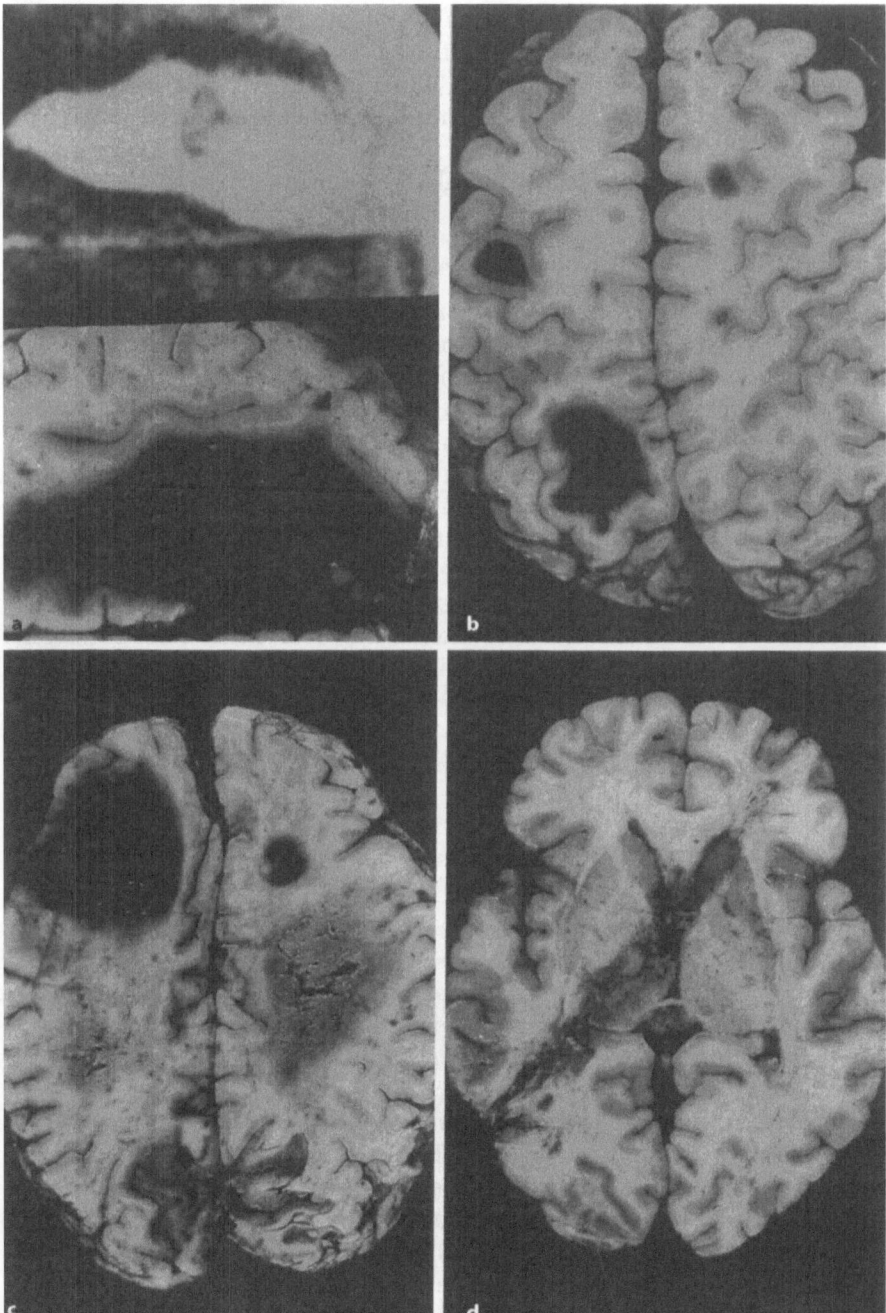

Fig. 3. a Laceration of the frontal region. Comparison between early CT scan and morphology. **b** Atypical symptomatic hemorrhages in the brain. Note localization of large and smaller bleeds. **c** Left, end-stage of traumatic hemorrhage; right, smaller hemorrhage. Mass shift from left to right by lateral infarction of the occipital region and consequent raised intracranial pressure. **d** Open head injury. Channel through the brain. In the right frontal region the channel leaves the plane of section

Some white matter hemorrhages may be situated next to midline structures other than the basal ganglia or pons. In traditional traumatic pathology such hemorrhages have been designated as "inner contusional foci" and have provoked efforts to explain their origin. In English they are now termed gliding contusions. Their localization permits their inclusion into the concept of primary axonal damage (see above, Fig. 2b).

Traumatic Epidural and Subdural Hemorrhage

Traumatic epidural hematoma is due to a rupture of a branch of a meningeal artery. For this to occur fracture of the skull is usually a prerequisite. Because of the anatomical situation of the "space" between the osseous and upper lamina of the dural structure, epidural hemorrhage tends to be more focally localized than subdural hemorrhage and occurs in more frontal, temporal or parieto-occipital regions.

In contrast, traumatic subdural hemorrhages are rather diffuse from the onset. They develop more or less dynamically, and different forms such as acute, subacute, and chronic can be distinguished clinically. We do not go into details here since the traumatic nature of a rapidly evolving subdural hematoma is beyond any doubt. It originates from the disruption of veins bridging the (virtual) subdural space. In hematomas that evolve slowly the connection with traumatic injury is often difficult to establish. In such cases minimal trauma must be assumed to be responsible, unless other mechnisms of origin exist. Overall it seems reasonable to include chronic subdural hematoma among the late (and therefore uncertain) sequelae of brain injury.

Open Head Injury

Open head injury is defined as a traumatic condition in which there is a direct connection between the spinal fluid and the environment. This connection facilitates the invasion of infectious material. By this definition, a nonmissile head injury would be classified as open if infection is possible. Basal skull fractures with liquorrhea to either nose or ear, however, have been considered by some authors as "intermediate" [24].

For the sake of simplicity, however, the term open head injury may be applied to replace the term "missile" head injury [1]. The cause of such an injury may be an object falling by accident or purposely propelled through the air (Fig. 3d). The impact and velocity of the missile dictates whether a depressed, penetrated, or perforated injury is sustained [12].

In depressed injuries the missile does not enter the brain but causes a fracture that by its inward dislocation causes contusions. Thus it is similar to a focal contusion, except for the open state. Penetrating objects remain partly or entirely within the nervous substance. The pathological feature is of hemorrhagic necrosis around the missile channel. The length of the channel and extent of necrosis depend upon a variety of factors such as the size and shape of the missile and its point of entry into the cranial vault. Perforating missiles, usually bullets, enter the skull through a relatively small hole but exit through a larger hole. Likewise, necrotic and hemorragic tissue develops along the wound channel. There is an increased risk of infection and epilepsy, in the all too seldom cases of bullet injury that are survived.

The Question of Direct and Delayed Conditions: Prospects

There are two concepts that are only partly consistent. The classical teaching holds that there may be a primary threefold damage with early and late consequences. The more recent notion distinguishes focal and generalized injury, the latter being either primary (DAI) or secondary. The main difference consists in the shift in prognostic implication. If it is true that DAI is underestimated and irreversible, then neuroprotection to prevent secondary damage would be useless to a large extent. The occurrence and mechanism of diffuse axonal injury has been confirmed successfully by experiments and has gained increasing attention during the past decade. Adams [1] has stressed repeatedly the importance of this pathogenetic principle for the explanation of unsolved questions in neurotraumatology. However, the concept is far from obtaining general acceptance. Authors who retain the conventional interpretation argue that the diffuse axonal damage with the sequence of histologically demonstrable findings of retraction balls and glial scars has been documented in few human cases only [22]. On the other hand, contusional cortical and hemorrhagic injuries are by no means seldom and are largely accepted both in neuropathology and forensic pathology. Thus DAI even in some recent extensive compilations of traumatic damage to the nervous system plays only a marginal role [22].

There seems to be one handicap for the common acceptance of DAI: the difficulty of its exact demonstration, which requires histological and even special neurohistological methods. The situation has, however, changed very recently. It has been claimed that immunohistochemistry now allows a much more comprehensive and rapid recognition of this traumatic condition. Antibodies against neurofilament proteins and ubiquitin have been used to demonstrate the axonal injury. The marker character of APP, amyloid precursor protein, has most recently been put forward [5, 9]. The detection of those markers is possible even in archived, conventionally treated material [15]. With these recent results in hand, the holders of the DAI hypothesis now underscore the earlier assumption that the diffuse axonal injury has been underestimated; it seems to be the usual mechanism of any traumatic event in the nervous system that is sufficiently severe [8].

To come to a general acceptance of either pathogenetic concept, systematic prospective studies are yet lacking. They could equally shed new light upon the questions of late sequelae of brain injury such as Bollinger's delayed apoplexia [23], various forms of postraumatic epilepsies, and the not yet completely solved question of traumatic causation of neoplastic growth [25].

References

1. Adams JH (1992) Head injury. In: Adams JH, Duchen, LW (eds) Grenfield's neuropathology 5th edn. Arnold, London
2. Adams JH, Graham DI, Murray S, Scott G (1982) Diffuse axonal injury due to non missile head injury in humans: an analysis of 45 cases. Ann Neurol 12: 537–563
3. Adams JH, Doyle D, Graham DI, Laurence AE, McLellan DR (1986) Gliding contusion in non-missile head injury in humans. Arch Pathol Lab Med 110: 485–488
4. Bähr M, Eschweiler GW, Dichgans J (1994) Neuronale Protektion bei neurologischen Erkrankungen? Nervenarzt 65: 355–360
5. Blumbergs PC, Scott, G, Manavis J, Wainwright, H, Simpson DA, McLean, AJ (1994) Staining of amyloid precursor protein to study axonal damage in mild head injury. Lancet 344: 1055–1056
6. Cajal S, Ramon I (1959) Degeneration and regeneration of the nervous system, vol. 2. Hafner, New York
· 7. Delank HW (1988) Das gedeckte Schädel-Hirn-Trauma – neurologische Aspekte. In: Das Gehirn und seine Erkrankungen (II) Graul EH, Pütter S, Loew D (Hrsg) MEDICENALE XVIII, Iserlohn
8. Gentleman SM, Roberts GW, Gennarelli TA, Maxwell WL, Adams JH, Kerr, S, Graham, DI (1995) Axonal injury: a universal consequence of fatal closed head injury? Acta Neuropathol (Berl) 89(6)537–543
9. Gultekin SH, Smith, TW (1994) Diffuse axonal injury in craniocerebral trauma. A comparative histologic and immunohistochemical study. Arch Pathol Lab Med 118(2)168–171
10. Kolisko A (1911) Über Gehirnruptur. Beiträge zur gerichtlichen Medizin. Deuticke, Leipzig
11. Krauland W (1950) Über Hirnschäden durch stumpfe Gewalt. Dtsch Zschr N 163: 265–328
12. Lindenberg R (1971) Trauma of meninges and brain. In: Minckler J (ed) Pathology of the nervous system, vol 2. McGraw Hill, New York
13. Schwarzacher W (1924) Über traumatische Markblutungen des Gehirns. Jahrbuch Psychiatr 43: 113
14. Sellier K, Unterharnscheidt F (1963) Mechanik und Pathomorphologie der Hirnschäden nach stumpfer Gewalteinwirkung auf den Schädel durch Windschutzscheiben. Hefte Unfallheilk 76
15. Sherriff FE, Bridges LR, Gentleman SM, Sivaloganathan S, Wilson S (1994) Markers of axonal injury in post mortem human brain. Acta Neuropathol (Berl) 88(5)433–439
16. Spatz H (1929) Kann man alte Rindendefekte traumatischer und arteriosklerotischer Genese voneinander unterscheiden? Die Bedeutung des "état vermolu." Arch Psychiatr 90: 885–887
17. Spatz H (1936) Pathologische Anatomie der gedeckten Hirnverletzungen mit besonderer Berücksichtiung der Rindenkontusion. Arch Psychiatr Nervenkr 105: 80–83
18. Strich SJ (1956) Diffuse degeneration of the cerebral white matter in severe dementia following head injury. J Neurol Neurosurg Psychiatr 19: 163–184
19. Strich SJ (1968) Notes on the marking method for staining degeneration myelin in the peripheral and central nervous system. J Neurol Neurosurg Psychatry 31: 110–114
20. Symonds CP (1962) Concussion and its sequelae. Lancet 1: 1–5
21. Symonds CP (1940) Concussion and contusion of the brain. In: Brook S (ed) Injuries of the skull, brain and spinal cord. Baillière, London, pp 71–115
22. Unterharnscheidt F (1993) Pathologie des Nervensystems VI.A-C, Traumatologie von Hirn und Rückenmark. In: Doerr W, Seifert G, Uehlinger E (eds) Spezielle Pathologische Anatomie, vol 13
23. Zülch KJ (1968) Zur Frage der posttraumatischen Spätapoplexie. In: Alemà E (ed) Brain and mind problems. A jubilee volume in honour of Prof. M. Gozzano. Il Pensiero Scientifico, Rome
24. Zülch KJ (1969) Pathologische Anatomie, Physiopathologie und Pathomechanismus des Schädelhirntraumas. Bull Soc Sci Méd Luxembourg 106: 153–211
25. Zülch KJ, Mennel HD (1971) Gehirntumor und Trauma. Hefte Unfallheilk 107: 33–44
26. Zülch KJ, Mennel HD, Zimmermann V (1974) Intracranial hypertension. In: Vinken PJ, Bruyn, GW (eds) Handbook of clinical neurology, vol 16. Tumors of the brain and skull. North Holland/Elsevier, Amsterdam, pp 89–149

4 Preclinical Emergency Management of Severe Brain Injuries and Polytraumata

P. Sefrin and C. Apfel

Despite the decline of severe traffic accidents in the emergency service the proportion of brain injuries and polytraumata has not decreased. The reason for this lies in the increase in accidents in the household and during leisure activities. While in the past many of these patients died immediately at the place of accident or during transport, today more patients reach the clinic due to earlier initiation and higher quality of medical care in the emergency service. Today the standard of preclinical management in Germany includes a medical physician specially qualified in emergency medicine.

Although polytraumata and brain injuries as a consequence of exogenic forces displays two different patterns of trauma, they have in common the acute vital threat due to hypoxemia and hypotension as well as their resulting secondary complications, which may have their roots in preclinical management and may limit subsequent intensive care therapy. Therefore the focus lies on the preclinical treatment of respiratory and cardial impairments. This may be difficult if there is no direct access possible, for example, in patients intercalated in a car, and if symptoms of respiratory or cardiac impairments are lacking. In patients with severe brain injuries the cardinal symptom of loss of consiousness leads to the adequate management. This is in contrast to a patient with a polytrauma, especially if he is young, since endogenous compensating mechanisms may result in a discrepancy for a longer period between the intensity of the trauma and recognizable vital impairments masking the need for early and aggressive therapy.

Despite a standardized first therapy in the preclinical area it is not always possible to stop early pathophysiological changes, and thus complications such as a multiorgan failure still occur. The polytrauma initiates imflammatory processes, where numerous humoral and cellular mediator and cascades systems are activated, leading to a self-perpetuating circle. The common mechanism is the impairment of terminal divisions leading to insufficient perfusion of vital organs. Pathophysiological consequences are a result of combination of organ and tissue trauma, massive liberation of catecholamins, and mediators and the hypovolemic shock. Precondition of a successful therapy of the partly selfperpetuating impairments is not only the early initiation of shock therapy but, if possible – the removal of the initiating cause and the discontinuation of the impairments due to the shock mechanisms itself.

The preclinical concept of care works stepwise, with the extention of therapy adjusted to the patient's general condition and the duration until clinical therapy can be performed (i. e., length of transport). Preclinical management is also affected by logistic problems such as access to the patient, the possibility of assessment, the duration and extention of the preclinical care, and the duration of transport to hospital. The main point is to stabilize or restitute respiratory and cardiac function. Hypotension and hypoxemia are the main causes of secondary impairments in patients with brain injuries. Although all parts of Germany are covered by an ambulance system, therapy is often not sufficient since the resulting trauma is not clearly recognizable. To avoid cerebral ischemic secondary complications a perfusion pressure of 70 mm Hg is essential, since complications may develop within a few minutes. This means that the mean arterial pressure must remain at least 90 mm Hg. Impairments of vital functions may be caused by both causes of trauma.

In the case of the combined polytrauma and brain injury the problem of the priority of preclinical management arises during the first stage of resuscitation. The four principles that must be applied are discussed below.

Restitution and Stabilization of Oxygenation

Adjuvant application of oxygen is necessary to assure sufficient oxygenation during spontaneous ventilation. Early intubation and ventilation is the primary object of preclinical management in patients with brain injuries suffering deep unconsciousness and resulting respiratory insufficiency. The indication for intubation is evident to any emergency physician when the Glasgow Coma Scale is 8 points or less. However, this value does not represent a sharp cutoff since patients with better neurological status and simultaneous severe injuries in the face may show a rapid deterioration of ventilation so that early intubation may be indicated. The intubation is primarily performed orally and in case of a polytrauma without unconsciousness enabled by general anesthesia. For preclinical anesthesia numerous concepts exist, none of which has proven itself clearly the best. Therefore the choice of anesthesia depends on the experience of each emergency physician. For the choice of the anesthetic drugs in patients with brain injuries one should consider the way in which intracranial pressure, cerebral blood flow, cerebral blood volume and cerebral metabolism are affected [1]. Both hypnotic and sedative drugs must be administered according to their clinical effect since an otherwise adequate dosage may result in hypotension, especially in hypovolemic patients such as polytraumatic patients. Conventional hypnotics such as etomidate, methohexitone, and thiopentone do not raise intracranial pressure but may produce a drop in blood pressure. As an alternative in polytrauma without brain injury ketamine can be used for induction. It should not be used in combined brain injuries since ketamine leads to an increase in cerebral blood flow, regional brain metabolism, and intracranial pressure.

Despite numerous studies confirming the value of early intubation and ventilation [4] there are still difficulties on the part of the emergency physician in anesthetizing, intubating, and ventilating a spontaneously ventilating patient. The use of a moderate PEEP does not conflict with a brain injury but should be used as a protection.

Oxygenation should be monitored in ambulance service by pulsoxymeter and be kept higher than 95%. If ventilation is necessary, an additional capnometer may be useful, although this monitoring cannot currently be presumed to be available in the ambulance service. The prophylactic hyperventilation may aggravate cerebral ischemia and is therefore no longer compulsory in preclinical medicine.

Restitution and Stabilization of Circulation

Of equal importance as the early and sufficient oxygenation is the support or restitution of adequate systemic blood pressure. Early fluid therapy is indisputably the essential precondition to combat resulting perfusion impairments with subsequent decrease in oxygen supply. The goal of shock therapy is therefore the normalization or improvement of circulation, which includes both cardiac output and intravasal volume. This includes hemostasis of open wounds and the immobilization of fractures, especially of large tubular bones but also of instable dislocated pelvic fractures. The quantity of the volume to be applied in the preclinical service depends on the intensity of trauma, loss of blood, duration of shock, and age of the patient. In contrast to the possibilities in a hospital, the emergency physician is restricted to rather crude assessments without data from exact measurements. Global values such as pulse and blood pressure are only a rough guide.

The ideal solution for infusion is still a question of debate, although it is known that the rate of patients with adult respiratory distress syndrome is higher after the administration of cristalloid solutions only. In addition, the logistic problems of increased volume supply must be considered. For cristalline solutions 0.9% sodium chloride or Ringer's lactate solution can be used. Filling the intravasal volume doses requires doses three to four times larger than those with colloid solutions, which may result in temporary volume overload and pulmonary edema, especially in case of a capillary leakage or cerebral edema. Concerning colloid solutions hydroxyethyl starch (HES) is the gold standard in the preclinical therapy since dextrans may result in anaphylactic side effects, affect coagulation, and impair the renal function. Rather, gelatine solutions are used to bridge brief hypovolemic episodes in the clinic due to their relatively short half-life. Of the various HES preparations the more concentrated HES (6%) with a molecular weight of 200 kDa is generally used because of the stronger effect on the increase in the intravasal volume. Despite of the superiority of HES solutions one cannot avoid the additional use of cristalloid solutions to fill up the extracellular space, and a ratio of colloid to cristalloid solution of 2 to 1 has proven worthwhile in preclinical management [2].

It must be mentioned that hypertone/hyperoncotic solutions (e.g., 7.5 % sodium chloride combined with 10 % HES solution) have the advantage of a pronounced short effect (onset after 1–2 min) on the intravasal volume, the hemodynamics, and the regional blood flow after the administration of even small volumes (4 ml/kg) [3]. This is explained by the fast intravasal influx from the microvascular endothelium, the erythrocytes and the interstitial tissue [2]. Hypertonic solutions are undergoing clinical assessment for possible positive effects in patients with brain injuries.

Clinical experiences with aggressive volume therapy have led to the adoption of this approach for preclinical therapy. The dose of volume blood pressure is the only parameter, and therefore the substitution can be only approximate. It must be stressed that hemorrhagic shock is basically not caused by an isolated brain injury and principally indicates an extracranial cause for bleeding. If a stabilization of the blood pressure with volume therapy is not possible under preclinical conditions, prompt transport to hospital for operative hemostasis is justified; however a detailed information should be arranged in advance.

Analgesia and Sedation

Pain perception can present an aggravating factor of pathophysiological changes due to the extended trauma. For this reason, and not only as a comfort for the patient, a special analgesia and in ventilated patients an adequate sedation is absolutely necessary. Arterial hypertension is known to occur, especially after brain injuries. The reason is a hyperdynamic reaction caused by sympathetic stimulation which in turn leads to increased intracranial pressure. Therefore the therapeutic consequence is not the administration of an antihypertensive drug but the institution of sufficient pain management. Due to the high pain intensity opioids are the primary choice and are adminstered according to the clinical requirements. Even a small overdosage may well lead to hypotension, especially in hypovolemic patients. Benzodiazepines are recommended for the sedation; fixed combination of drugs should be avoided.

Neuroprotective Drugs

For patients with brain injury the efficacy of special drugs (e.g., steroids, calcium antagonists, barbiturates, Tris buffer) has not been confirmed. The standardized application of mannitol to act as an osmodiuretic is not indicated in the preclinical stage.

After the standardized therapy of the vital functions the second priority is medical attention to single injuries. The patient is then transported to an appropriate hospital while emergency monitoring is continued. Only the wise sequence of several single steps of therapy ensures the highest chances of restitution and survival in these patients.

References

1. Cunitz G (1995) Die Erstversorgung des Schädel-Hirn-Trauma-Patienten. Anaesthesist 44: 369–391
2. Walz M, Schildhauer TA, Muhr G (1995) Neues in der klinischen Schocktherapie. Chirurg 66: 1040–1049
3. Mazzoni MC, Warnke KC, Arfors KE, Skalak TC (1994) Capillary hemodynamics in hemorrhagic shock and perfusion: In vivo and model analysis. Am J Physiol 267: 1928
4. Sefrin P, de Pay AW (1994) Frühzeitige Beatmung im Rettungsdienst bei Polytrauma. Notfallmed 10: 231–243

5 Preclinical Treatment of Patients With Severe Brain Injuries

J. Piek

Introduction

Approximately 50 % of patients with head injuries die either at the scene of the accident or on arrival at hospital [1], most of them from secondary insults to the already injured brain. Adequate prehospital care is crucial for these patients. The concept of preventable death was first defined by Van Wagoner [2] in 1961. Jennett and Carlin [3] referred specifically to patients with head injuries and noted that most preventable deaths from head injury are caused by inappropriate prehospital management. As early as 1958 MacIver et al. adressed the problem of prehospital hypoxia [4] and stated that "anoxia is the main cause of death in patients who survive the accident but die at a later stage." Recognizing that almost one-third of trauma deaths in nondesignated hospitals are preventable [5], the American College of Surgeons [6] and the Joint Section of Trauma of the American Association of Neurological Surgeons and the Congress of Neurological Surgeons have developed [7] criteria for designated (neuro-)trauma centers. Development of these specialized regional trauma centers has contributed enormously to improved survival and outcome for trauma patients.

In Germany a system of rapid-response trauma transportation ambulances equipped with advanced medical treatment crews and standardized technical equipment has been designed both to provide medical treatment at the site of any injury and to shorten transportation time to hospital. This has been followed by area-covering helicopters located at major trauma centers to cover larger distances. The medical effectiveness of this system has been demonstrated for multitrauma [8] and for head-injured [9] patients. Its cost-effectiveness has also been demonstrated [10].

The Role of Secondary Insults to the Brain

Emergency care of the patient with a severe brain injury is based on rapid and accurate diagnosis of the primary injury and early aggressive treatment and/or prevention of secondary insults. Extracranial complications are the main contributors to secondary brain damage in the preclinical phase. Hypotension and hypoxia play a major role as the acutely injured brain is especially susceptible to these insults [11].

Incidence of Secondary Insults

In large series of patients with traumatic brain injury (TBI) the incidence of prehospital *hypotension* varies from 12.2% to 34.6% [12–16], with a remarkable decline during the last 15 years (Fig. 1). Depending on the definition, hypoxemia is present in 30% [17] to 45.6% [18] of patients with severe head injuries. Even in patients with moderate head injuries the incidence of *hypoxemia* is as high as 14.8% [14]. In patients with severe injuries hypercarbia occurs in up to 6.1% [14]. Our own data show *hypocarbia* in 16.2% of patients (Fig. 2).

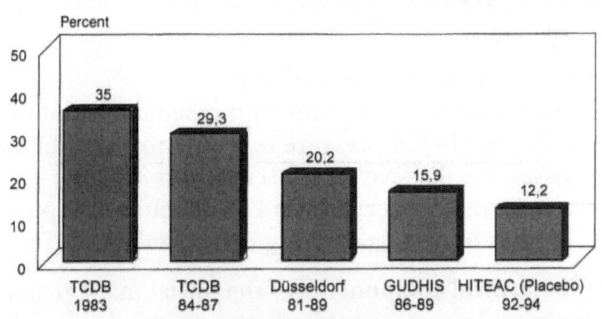

Fig. 1. Incidence of prehospital hypotension in patients with severe head injuries during the last 25 years (13–16)

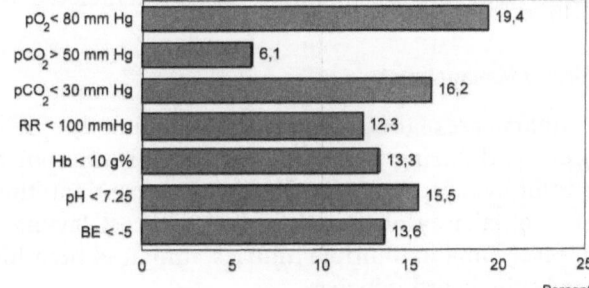

Fig. 2. Incidence of secondary insults in patients with severe head injuries (1136 patients with severe head injuries, 1981–1989: Neurosurgical Department, Heinrich Heine University, Düsseldorf)

Effect of Secondary Insults on Outcome

Extracranial complications occur frequently in severely head-injured patients. The effect of secondary insults on the outcome of patients with severe TBI has well been documented [3, 12, 17–26]. Although the outcome of an individual patient may be adversely affected by a number of different complications, only a few have been identified to have an independent effect on outcome. In addition to hypotension and hypoxia, these include pneumonia, septicemia, and coagulopathy [24]. When prehospital hypoxia and/or hypotension are present in patients with TBI, the mortality rate is at least doubled. Conversely, normotensive/normoxic patients are twice as likely to make a good recovery [12, 18, 19, 21].

In summary, it can be concluded that improvement of preclinical care of patients with severe head injuries reduces the incidence of secondary insults to the injured brain and further improves outcome in these patients. Intense training of the medical emergency crews and the physicians involved in the referring hospitals can improve the preclinical care for these patients.

Prevention of Secondary Insults

Assessment and stabilization of patients with head injuries begins at the scene of the injury by experienced emergency medical personal. This includes the following:

- Securing the patient's airway
- Maintaining oxygenation and normal ventilation
- Initiating blood pressure resuscitation and fluid administration
- Assessing the level of consciousness
- Stabilizing the cervical and thoracolumbar spine
- Identifying and stabilizing extracranial injuries

Other critical components of the initial management of such patients include obtaining information about the mechanism of the injury and providing a rapid transport to a qualified medical center.

Airway Management

Primary care of the patient with TBI is aimed at preserving a clear airway at the scene and during the entire transport. Numerous factors may cause hypoxia and/or hypercarbia in the head-injured patient: the influence of drugs and/or alcohol, airway obstruction due to direct laryngeal or pharyngeal trauma, chest trauma in multiple injuries, impaired breathing due to TBI, and associated spinal cord injuries.

Initial administration of oxygen (e.g., O_2: 6 l/min via face mask) is mandatory in all patients with a TBI. The risk of pneumonia increases with the presence of coma and with impairment of airway reflexes [27]. Intubation in patients with severe head injuries reduces the rate of aspiration and helps to prevent respiratory insuffiency [28]. Patients with a total Glasgow Coma Scale (GCS) [29] score no higher than 8 points or a GCS motor score below 5 points should be intubated and ventilated as soon as safely possible.

Intubation and ventilation should also be considered in patients with better scores and associated injuries that place them at the risk of acute hypoxia (e.g., severe maxillofacial injuries, thoracic trauma, high-level spinal cord injuries). Oral intubation should be preferred in the preclinical setting as nasotracheal intubation can lead to severe nasopharyngeal hemorrhage and subsequent aspiration [30]. With blind nasotracheal intubation there is also a small risk of transethmoidal perforation in patients with frontobasal fractures. During oral intubation the cervical spine should be stabilized manually in-line. Orotracheal intubation performed in this way has been shown to be safe without additional risk to exarcerbate a cervical cord injury [31]. Aspiration should be avoided and/or vigorously treated. Once a patient is intubated artificial ventilation should be performed. Our own experience shows that, in addition to not intubating a patient in whom intubation is indicated, the main cause for hypoxia in patients with head injuries is that intubated patients are allowed to breath spontaneously and are not ventilated [14]. Arterial saturation should be monitored by pulse oximetry [32]. Artificial ventilation should be adjusted to achieve an arterial saturation greater than 95%. It should be kept in mind that numerous factors such as hypothermia and shock affect the accuracy of this method (references in [33]). Aggressive hyperventilation should be avoided in the early phase of the injury when cerebral blood flow is typically at its lowest [34, 35]. If endtidal CO_2 can be measured, it should be kept between 30–35 mm Hg (= 4–4.66 kPa) in normotensive patients [36–38].

The importance of establishing a proper airway and providing adequate ventilation was shown in a study conducted in 1981–1989 at the Neurosurgical Department, Heinrich Heine University of Düsseldorf, on 1136 patients with severe head injuries. This study found P_aO_2 to be below 80 mm Hg in the following proportions of patients: 22.4% of those not intubated, 21.0% of those intubated and breathing spontaneously, and 16.0% of those intubated and ventilated.

Management of Blood Pressure and Circulation

Treatment of low blood pressure (BP) should aim at maintaining a cerebral perfusion pressure (CPP) of at least 60 mm Hg [39]. At least two large peripheral i. v. cannulas should be in place and secured with adhesive tape. The first step in establishing adequate cerebral perfusion pressure is establishing a normal BP. Treatment of low BP should aimed at maintaining systolic BP above 120 mm Hg (= 16 kPa) for adults. An increase in BP is usually caused by inadequate sedation and analgesia. If this is not the case, treatment of raised BP (> 200 mm Hg = 26.6 kPa) by vasoactive agents is usually not indicated and may cause fatal hypotension. It should be kept in mind that hypotension is rarely caused by an isolated head injury [17], and that the most common cause of this event is an extracranial injury (exception: newborns). As is well known, the combination of low BP and bradycardia often indicates neurogenic shock following spinal cord injuries at thoracic levels or higher.

Drugs

Volume Replacement. Adequate volume resuscitation should be initiated. Isotonic solutions (e. g., Ringer's solution, NaCl 0.9%) and colloids are advocated [40]. The i. v. administration of hypertonic saline increases systemic BP and cardiac output [41–45], but there is continuing debate whether hypertonic saline is superior in the acute resuscitative phase after head injury. Most animal models show a beneficial effect on intracranial pressure (ICP), brain water content, and hemodynamics [46 – 50], although cerebral oxygen delivery was not improved in an animal model of head injury and mild shock [51]. In the clinical setting case reports show a beneficial effect on ICP control [52 – 54], but prospective randomized studies are lacking. If given, hypertonic saline (250 cc NaCl 7.25 %) should be administered first, followed by rapid infusion of colloids. Hypotonic cristalloids (e. g., Glc 5 %, Ringer's lactate) may worsen cerebral edema [55].

Sedation/Analgesia. Adequate sedation and analgesia is essential in patients with head injuries, especially if ventilated. Sedatives and analgetics should be carefully titrated as overdosing may cause profound hypotension especially in hemodynamically unstable patients. Opioids combined with short-acting hypnotics can be used to facilitate the intubation procedure, the combination of an opioid and a short-acting benzodiazepine may be used for sedation during the transport.

Vasopressors. If volume replacement fails to assure an adequate systemic BP within minutes vasopressors should be considered. From a neurosurgical/neuroanesthetical point of view no vasopressor has been shown to be superior to others, subsequently no recommendations concerning the type of pressors can be given.

"Neuroprotective" Agents. Aside from numerous studies on so-called "neuroprotective" agents in the ICU treatment of severe head injuries, there are no prospective studies on the prehospital administration of such agents. During the 1970s and 1980s corticosteroids were widely used for the preclinical treatment of brain edema in Germany. Recent prospective, randomized trials, however, have shown no beneficial effects of high-dose corticosteroids in the acute phase of severe head injuries [15, 56].

Mannitol. Both experimental and clinical settings have shown mannitol to be effective in reducing ICP [57 – 63]. It expands the intravascular volume thus increasing systemic BP [57, 63]. As prospective trials for the prehospital period are lacking, its general use is not advocated during prehospital care. In emergency situations (dilating of a former narrow pupil), however, it can be administered (0.5 – 1 g/kg body weight with an infusion time of 10 – 15 min).

Transport

Monitoring. In Germany the monitoring equipment for ambulances is standardized (DIN EN 1789), both manual and automated indirect BP monitoring, pulse oximetry (DIN EN 865), stethoscope, thermometer, ECG monitoring. Respiratory monitoring for ventilated patients includes tidal volume, inspiratory O_2 concentration, airway pressure. Endtidal CO_2 should be monitored by capnography (DIN EN 864).

Patient. Although controversial [64, 65], the patient's head should be elevated at a 30° level. About 5%–10% of all head injury victims sustain a cervical spine injury [66–71]. A rigid collar should be applied as soon as possible to secure the cervical spine and kept in position until radiography shows beyond any doubt the absence of any cervical spine lesion down to the second thoracic vertebra. The spine should always lie in a neutral position on a rigid plate. In multiple-trauma patients unstable fractures of the limbs should be immobilized. Rolled sheets, sandbags, or commercially available devices should secure the position of the head. Endotracheal tubes should be secured by tapes, avoiding passing the tape around the neck not to compromise jugular venous return. After removing clothes, the patient should be carefully checked for further injuries. Of particular importance are thoracic, abdominal, pelvic, and limbic injuries, which carry a high risk for hypotension and/or hypoxemia. As experimental and clinical studies suggest the beneficial effect of mild hypothermia on cerebral edema formation [72–75], the patient's temperature should be kept at levels of mild hypothermia up to normothermia (34°–36°C).

Stretcher/Trolley. A complete system of transport with the patient "packed" together with monitoring and therapeutic devices is very useful. The patient should be positioned on a stretcher that allows intrahospital radiological imaging (RX, CT) so that it is the same from the scene until admission to the ward/ICU/OR.

Transportation Team. In addition to the driver (transport and communication), at least two persons should be responsible for the patients care. One of the team members should be a physician. Members of the team should be very familiar with the equipment and personally perform the daily checking of it. They should have received a specific training in: (a) airway care and tracheal intubation, (b) ventilation by mask and portable mechanical ventilator, (c) peripheral and central vein access, and (d) neurological examination of unconscious patients (see guidelines of the German Interdisciplinary Association of Critical Care Medicine, DIVI [76])

Neurological Assessment and Documentation

A complete and comprehensive chart should be compiled by the transporting team. A protocol should be used that is standardized at least regionally. For Germany the DIVI protocol [76] is widely accepted. The chart should contain additional copies to provide the information to the referring hospitals. Documentation should include information (minimum) on:

- Patient's name, sex, address, birthdate
- Time, nature, cause of the injury

- Medical history (if possible)
- Neurological state: GCS [29] score (broken into eye, verbal and motor), pupil reactivity, focal neurological deficits
- Extracranial injuries
- Trauma score (standardized at least on a regional level)
- Repeated documentation of pulse, BP; SO_2, endtidal CO_2 (if possible)
- Administered medication (type, dose, timing)
- Interventions (type, timing)
- Free space for comments
- Name and telephone number of the transporting physician

Advance radio communication of the patient's clinical status to the receiving hospital medical staff is strongly advocated and requires standard local guidelines.

Feedback and Quality Assessment

After delivery of the patient members of the hospital medical staff should compile a form containing any observation (especially problems) related to the trasferral of the patient. This form (standardized at least at a regional level) should be given to the transporting team to assure quality of the patients transport. Regional conferences should be held on a regular basis between emergency teams and the receiving hospitals to assure and improve the quality of prehospital care. Guidelines by the national organizations involved in the prehospital care of head trauma patients may further improve preclinical care of such patients [77, 78].

References

1. Klauber MR, Marshall LF, Toole BM (1985) Cause of decline in head-injured mortality rate in San Diego County. J Neurosurg 62: 528–531
2. Van Wagoner FH (1961) Died in hospital: a three-year study of deaths following trauma. J Trauma 1: 401–408
3. Jennett B, Carlin J (1978) Preventable mortality and morbidity after head injury. Injury 10: 31–39
4. MacIver IN, Frew IJC, Matheson JG (1958) The role of respiratory insufficiency in the mortality of severe head injuries. Lancet 1: 390–393
5. Cales RH, Trunkey DD (1985) Preventable trauma deaths: a review of trauma care systems development. JAMA 254: 1059–1063
6. Committee on Trauma (1986) Hospital and prehospital resources for the care of the injured patient. Bull Am Coll Surg 71: 4–12
7. Pitts LH, Ojemann RG, Quest DO (1987) Neurotrauma care and the neurosurgeon: A statement from the Joint Section of Trauma of the AANS and CNS. J Neurosurg 67: 783–785
8. Schmidt U, Herlich M, Frame SB et al (1991) On-scene helicopter transport of the multitrauma patient – comparison of a German and an American system. J Trauma 31: 1038
9. Colohan ART, Alves WM, Gross CR et al (1989) Head injury mortality in two centers with different emergency medical services and intensive care. J Neurosurg 71: 202–207
10. Deutscher Verkehrssicherheitsrat, Bayerisches Staatsministerium des Inneren (1985) Not-

fallrettung Unterfranken. Zur Wirksamkeit und Wirtschaftlichkeit des Rettungsdienstes. Dokumentation II (Internal publication by the ministry of health)
11. Jenkins LW, Mosszynski K, Lyeth BF et al (1989) Increased vulnerability of the mildly traumatized rat brain to cerebral ischemia: the use of controlled secondary ischemia as a research tool to identify common or different mechanisms contributing to mechnical and ischemic brain injury. Brain Res 477: 211–224
12. Marshall LF, Becker DP, Bowers SA et al (1983) The National Traumatic Coma Data Bank. I. Design, purpose, goals, and results. J Neurosurg 59: 276–284
13. Chesnut RM, Marshall SB, Piek J et al (1993) Early and late systemic hypotension as a frequent and fundamental source of cerebral ischemia following severe brain injury in the Traumatic Coma Data Bank. Acta Neurochir Suppl (Wien) 59: 121–125
14. Wahjoepramono EJ, Piek J, Bock WJ (1993) prehospital airway care and control of ventilation in patients with head injuries – a retrospective analysis in 1623 head trauma victims. In: Lorenz R, Brock M, Klinger M (eds) Advances in neurosurgery 21. Springer, Berlin Heidelberg New York, pp 184–187
15. Gaab MR and the German GUDHIS Study Group (1995) Ultrahohe Dexamethason-Gabe beim akuten Schädelhirntrauma. Ergebnisse einer prospektiven randomisierten Doppelblind-Multicenter-Studie (GUDHIS). Zbl Neurochir 55: 135–143
16. Marshall LF (ND) Results from the protocol P-2700-0036 (Tirilazad in patients with moderate and severe head injuries). (unpublished)
17. Miller JD, Sweet RC, Narayan RK et al (1978) Early insult to the injured brain. JAMA 240: 439–442
18. Chesnut RM, Marshall LF, Klauber MR et al (1993) The role of secondary brain injury in determining outcome from severe head injury. J Trauma 34: 216–222
19. Wald SL, Shackford SR, Fenwick J (1993) The effect of secondary insults on mortality and long-term disability after severe head injury in a rural region without a trauma system. J Trauma 34: 377–381
20. Bowers SA, Marshall LF (1980) Outcome in 200 consecutive cases of severe head injury in San Diego County: a prospective analysis. Neurosurgery 6: 237–242
21. Miller JD, Becker DP (1982) Secondary insults to the injured brain. J R Coll Surg Edinb 27: 292–298
22. Klauber MR, Marshall LF, Luerssen TG et al (1989) Determinants of head injury mortality: Importance of the low risk patient. Neurosurgery 24: 31–36
23. Newfield P, Pitts L, Kaktis J et al (1980) The influence of shock on mortality after head trauma. Crit Care Med 8: 254
24. Piek J, Chesnut RM, Marshall LF et al (1992) Extracranial complications of severe head injury. J Neurosurg 77: 901–907
25. Price DJE, Murray A (1972) Influence of hypoxia and hypotension on recovery from head injury. Injury 3: 218–224
26. Rose J, Valtonen S, Jennett B (1977) Avoidable factors contributing to death after head injury. BMJ 21: 615–618
27. Chevret S, Hemmer M, Carlet J et al (1993) Incidence and risk factors of pneumonia acquired in intensive care units. Results from a multicenter prospective study on 996 patients. European Cooperative Group on Nosocomial Pneumonia. Intensive Care Med 19: 256–264
28. Singbartl G (1985) Die Bedeutung der präklinischen Notfallversorgung für die Prognose von Patienten mit schwerem Schädel-Hirn-Trauma. Anaesth Intensivther Notfallmed 20: 251–260
29. Teasdale G, Jennett B (1976) Assessment of coma after head injury. Acta Neurochir (Wien) 34: 45–55
30. Tintinelli JE, Claffey J (1981) Complications of nasotracheal intubation. Ann Emerg Med 10: 142–144
31. Rhee KJ, Green W, Holcroft JW et al (1990) Oral intubation in the multiply injured patient: the risk of exacerbating spinal cord damage. Ann Emerg Med 19: 45–48
32. Silverstone P (1989) Pulse oximetry at the roadside: a study of pulse oximetry in immediate care. BMJ 298: 711–713
33. Curley JF, Smyrnios NA (1991) Routine monitoring of the critically ill: In: Rippe JM, Irwin RS, Alpert JS, Fink MP (eds) Intensive care medicine. Little Brown, Boston, pp 199–214

34. Bouma GJ, Muizelaar JP, Stringer A et al (1992) Ultraearly evaluation of regional cerebral blood flow in severely head-injured patients using xenon-enhanced computerized tomography. J Neurosurg 77: 360–368
35. Obrist WD, Marion DW, Aggarwal S (1993) Time course of cerebral blood flow and metabolic changes following severe head injury. Abstracts, 61st Annual Meeting of The American Neurological Surgeons, Boston, April
36. Gopinath SP, Robertson CS, Contant CF et al (1994) Jugular venous desaturationand outcome after head injury. Psychiatry Neurosci 57: 717–723
37. Muizelar JP, Marmarou A, Ward JD et al (1991) Adverse effects of prolonged hyperventilation in patients with severe head injury: A randomized clinical trial. J Neurosurg 75: 731–739
38. Van Helden A, Schneider GH, Unterberg A et al (1993) Monitoring of jugular venous oxygen saturation as a guide to therapy in severe head injury. Abstracts, 2nd International Neurotrauma Symposium, Glasgow, July
39. Kiening KL, Unterberg AW, Bardt TF et al (1996) Monitoring of cerebral oxygenation in patients with severe head injuries: brain tissue PO2 versus jugular vein oxygen saturation. J Neurosurg 85: 751–757
40. College of Surgeons (1989) Advanced trauma life support course. College of Surgeons, Chicago
41. Valesco IT, Potieri Y, Rocha e Silva M et al (1980) Hypertonic NaCl and severe hemorrhagic shock. Am J Physiol 239: 664–673
42. Nakayama S, Sibley L, Gunther RA et al (1984) Small volume resuscitation with hypertonic saline (2400 mOsmol/l) during hemorrhagic shock. Circ Shock 13: 149–159
43. Rocha e Silva M, Negraes GA et al (1986) Hypertonic resuscitation from severe hemorrhagic shock: patterns of regional circulation. Circ Shock 19: 165–175
44. Meniga PA, Mattox KL, Pepe PE et al (1989) Hypertonic saline-dextrane solutions for the prehospital management of traumatic hypotension. Am J Surg 157: 528–534
45. Vassar MJ, Perry CA, Gannaway WL et al (1991) 7,5 % sodium chloride/dextran for resuscitation of trauma patients undergoing helicopter transport. Arch Surg 126: 1065–1072
46. Freshman SP, Battistella FD, Matteucci M et al (1993) Hypertonic saline (7.5 %) versus mannitol: a comparison for treatment of acute head injuries. J Trauma 35: 344–348
47. Berger S, Schürer L, Hartl R et al (1994) 7.2 % NaCl/10 % dextran 60 versus 20 % mannitol for treatment of intracranial hypertension. Acta Neurochir Suppl (Wien) 60: 494–498
48. Berger S, Schürer L, Hartl R et al (1995) Reduction of post-traumatic intracranial hypertension by hypertonic/hyperoncotic saline/dextran and hypertonic mannitol. Neurosurgery 37: 98–107
49. Taylor G, Myers S, Kurth CD et al (1996) Hypertonic saline improves brain resuscitation in a pediatric model of head injury and hemorrhagic shock. J Pediatr Surg 31: 65–70
50. Sheikh AA, Matsuoka T, Wisner DH (1996) Cerebral effects of resuscitation with hypertonic saline and a new low-sodium hypertonic fluid in hemorrhagic shock and head injury. Crit Care Med 24: 1226–1232
51. DeWitt DS, Prough DS, Deal DD et al (1996) Hypertonic saline does not improve cerebral oxygen delivery after head injury and mild hemorrhage in cats. Crit Care Med 24: 109–117
52 Gunnar WD, Merlotti GJ, Jonasson O et al (1986) Resuscitation from hemorrhagic shock: alterations of the intracranial pressure after normal saline, 3 % saline and dextran 40. Ann Surg 204: 686–692
53. Worthley LIG, Cooper DJ, Jones N (1988) Treatment of resistant intracranial hypertension with hypertonic saline. J Neurosurg 68: 478–481
54. Holcroft JW, Vassar MJ, Turner JE et al (1987) Three percent NaCl and 7.5 % NaCl-dextran in the resuscitation of severely head-injured patients. Ann Surg 206: 279–288
55. Tommasino C, Moore S, Todd MM (1988) Cerebral effects of isovolemic hemodilution with cristalloid or colloid solutions. Crit Care Med 16: 862–868
56. Grumme Th, Baethmann A, Kolodziejczyk D et al (1995) Treatment of patients with severe head injury by triamcinolone: a prospective, controlled multicenter clinical trial of 396 cases. Res Exp Med 195: 217–229
57. Wise BL, Chater ML (1962) The value of hypertonic mannitol solution in decreasing brain mass and lowering cerebro-spinal pressure. J Neurosurg 19: 1038–1043
58. Shenkin HA, Goluboff B, Haft H (1962) The use of mannitol for the reduction of intracranial pressure in intracranial surgery. J Neurosurg 19: 897–901

59. McQueen JD, Jeanes LD (1964) Dehydration and rehydration of the brain with hypertonic urea and mannitol. J Neurosurg 21: 1–8
60. Miller JD, Leech P (1975) Effects of mannitol and steroid therapy on intracranial volume-pressure relationships in patients. J Neurosurg 42: 274–281
61. Cottrell JE, Robustelli A, Post K et al (1977) Furosemide- and mannitol-induced changes in intracranial pressure and serum osmolarity and electrolytes. Anesthesiology 47: 28–30
62. Muizelaar JP, Lutz HA III, Becker DP (1984) Effect of mannitol on ICP and CBF and correlation with pressure autoregulation in severely head-injured patients. J Neurosurg 61: 700–706
63. Rosner MJ, Coley I (1987) Cerebral perfusion pressure: a hemodynamic mechanism of mannitol and the postmannitol hemogram. Neurosurgery 21: 147–156
64. Feldman Z, Kanter M, Robertson CS et al (1992) Effect of head elevation on intracranial pressure, cerebral perfusion pressure, and cerebral blood flow in head-injured patients. J Neurosurg 76: 207–211
65. Rosner MJ, Coley IB (1986) Cerebral perfusion pressure, intracranial pressure, and head elevation. J Neurosurg 65: 636–641
66. Jennett B, Teasdale G, Galbraith S et al (1977) Severe head injury in three countries. J Neurol Neurosurg Psychiatr 40: 291–298
67. Miller JD, Butterworth JF, Gudeman SK et al (1981) Further experience in the management of severe head injury. J Neurosurg 54: 289–299
68. Gentleman D, Teasdale G, Murray L (1986) Cause of severe head injury and risk of complications. BMJ 292: 449–453
69. Moskopp D, Böker KD, Kurthen M et al (1990) Begleitende Wirbelsäulentraumata bei Schädel-Hirn-Verletzten. Unfallchirurg 93: 120–126
70. Pagni CA, Massaro F (1991) Concomitant cranio-cerebral and vertebro-medullary injuries. Analysis of 121 cases. Acta Neurochir 111: 1–10
71. Hills MW, Deane SA (1993) Head Injury and facial injury: is there an increased risk of cervical spine injury? J Trauma 34: 549–554
72. Busto R, Globus MY, Dietrich WD et al (1989) Effect of mild hypothermia on ischemia-induced release of neurotransmitters and free fatty acids in rat brain. Stroke 20: 904–910
73. Marion DW, Obrist WD, Carlier PM (1993) The use of moderate therapeutic hypothermia for patients with severe head injuries: a preliminary report. J Neurosurg 79: 354–362
74. Shiozaki T, Sugimoto H, Taneda M (1993) Effect of mild hypothermia on uncontrollable intracranial hypertension after severe head injury. J Neurosurg 79: 363–368
75. Clifton GL, Allen S, Barrodale P et al (1993) A phase II study of moderate hypothermia in severe brain injury. J Neurotrauma 10: 263–271
76. Deutsche Interdisziplinäre Vereinigung für Intensiv- und Notfallmedizin (DIVI) (1995) Stellungnahmen, Empfehlungen zu Problemen der Intensiv- und Notfallmedizin, 3rd edn, Asmuth, Cologne
77. Bullock R, Chesnut RM, Clifton G et al (1996) Guidelines for the management of severe head injury. J Neurotrauma 13: 639–734
78. Working Group "Neurosurgical Intensive Care/Neurotraumatology" of The German Socitey for Neurosurgery, Working Group "Neuroanaesthesia" of the German Society for Anaesthesiology and Intensive Care Medicine (1996) Guidelines for the prehospital care of patients with head injuries. Mitteilungen der Deutschen Gesellschaft für Neurochirurgie 4

6 The Traumatic Carotid Cavernous Fistula: Clinical Features, Diagnosis, and Therapy

S. Bien and J.P. Wakat

Introduction

Three types of carotid artery-cavernous sinus fistulae have to be distinguished:

1. Dural external and internal carotid artery-cavernous sinus fistulae
2. Direct, spontaneous, internal carotid artery-cavernous fistulae, and
3. Direct, traumatic internal carotid artery-cavernous fistulae

In this article we will discuss only the last of the three. Traumatic carotid cavernous fistulae (TCCFs) occur as a result of a major head trauma with direct or indirect traumatization of the head. Car accidents are a common cause of a TCCF, but direct impact with pointed or blunt force (e. g., domestic accidents) can lead to a TCCF. The trauma has to be adequately severe; minor traumas normally do not result in a rupture of the internal carotid artery and the occurence of a TCCF. The latter can also occur postoperatively after various surgical interventions [5, 26, 30 a].

Clinical Appearance

The specific clinical symptomatology of TCCFs is uniform, but it has to be differentiated from symptoms of accompanying injury (e. g., epidural hematoma, acute subdural hematoma). An isolated TCCF displays chemosis as a prelimi-

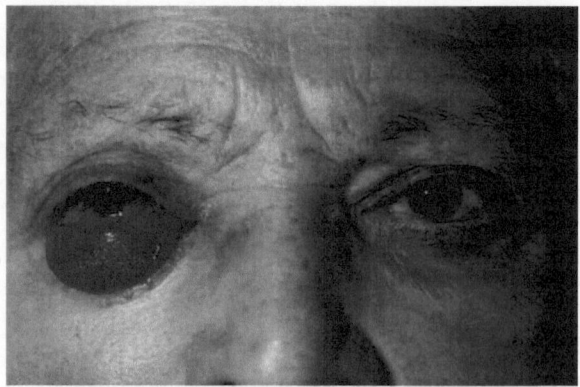

Fig 1. Severe chemosis and ophthalmoplegia in a 78-year-old female with a right sided TCCF

nary symptom (Fig. 1), sometimes even to a great extent. If the patient has not lost consciousness as a result of the trauma, he or she can usually hear a pulsatile and auscultatable noise from a postorbital direction. Further analysis reveals an impairment of the ocular muscles or even complete ophthalmoplegia. As a secondary symptom visual disturbance can appear as a result of venous congestion or increased intra-ocular pressure. These symptoms develop either directly after traumatization or after a few days of latency.

The patient is at risk for several reasons: the homolateral eye (or, in cases with bilateral venous drainage, both eyes) suffers from venous congestion; patients with an insufficient circle of Willis are at risk of cerebral hypoperfusion; the venous overload can cause elevated cerebral pressure; and when cerebral veins are involved int the drainage, they may rupture and cause an intracranial hemorrhage.

Etiology and Hemodynamics

The TCCF arises from a direct traumatization of the internal carotid artery within its cavernous course. The rupture is typically of macroscopic size; the shunt volume is always very high. It has a dramatic hemodynamic influence on the hemisphere beyond the rupture (Fig. 2a). In patients with large fistulae, the enormous shunt volume does not allow any blood supply from intracranial circulation beyond the fistula site. Flow phenomena with steal from the intracranial internal carotid artery and from the vertebrobasilar circulation might develop and yield to secondary neurologic deficits due to the reduced blood supply.

Therapy

Due to possible severe cerebral or ophthalmological complications, the TCCF should be treated as a relative emergency, especially when angiography findings (pseudoaneurysms, large venous pouches, drainage into cortical veins) show a fistula of higher risk [20, 32].

The intracavernous section of the carotid artery is not very accessible to surgery, especially in the case of traumatized carotids with high-flow fistulae towards the cavernous sinus. Therefore a real therapeutic alternative to interventional neuroradiology does not exist. An early attempt at therapy consisted in a surgical ligature of the internal carotid artery outside the cavernous sinus (cervical and/or intracranial) [22]. If the fistula itself is not occluded completely, anastomoses via the circle of Willis or the opthalmic artery will revasculize the fistula quite often. Consequently an unselective occlusion of the internal carotid artery – distant from the fistula – has to be considered as contraindicated. Even short-term improvement is not a sufficient reason for such a therapy. In addition to this a ligation of the internal carotid artery with the fistula obstructs or even prevents subsequent adequate endovascular therapy, because direct access through the ligated artery is then no longer feasible.

The introduction of balloon catheters allowed the occlusion of the fistula and the carrying carotid artery, which lead to a noticeable improvement of the prognosis [28, 29]. However the introduction of detachable balloons by Debrun et al. in the 1970s finally allowed a definitive and carotid artery preserving therapy of TCCFs [7 – 11].

Via conventional transfemoral access a balloon catheter is placed inside the carotid artery and guided by blood flow towards the fistula mund. By inflating the balloon, it is aspirated into the high-flow fistula. And by being inflated, it occludes the fistula from outside the carotid artery [1, 2, 6, 12, 14, 15, 23, 24]. Occasionally, several balloons are needed for a complete occlusion of the fistula. Mild to moderate stenosis is of no clinical importance. The internal carotid artery usually can be kept patent [3]. Cicatrization of the fistula takes place within a few weeks; subsequent leaking of the balloon is meaningless. Routine examinations reveal pseudo-aneurysms located at the deflated balloons, which do not need any further treatment.

Several therapeutic alternatives remain, if selective occlusion of the fistula under preservation of the internal carotid artery does not succeed. After a tolerance test the TCCF itself and the accompanying internal carotid artery can both be occluded by using a large balloon. But the occlusion of the fistula itself is indispensable, as late occurrences are possible if the fistula is left open and the internal carotid artery is occluded proximal to the fistula [13]. The procedure cannot always be tolerated by the patient and implies an incalculable risk of future cerebral complications. In our own series [3], we tried to avoid

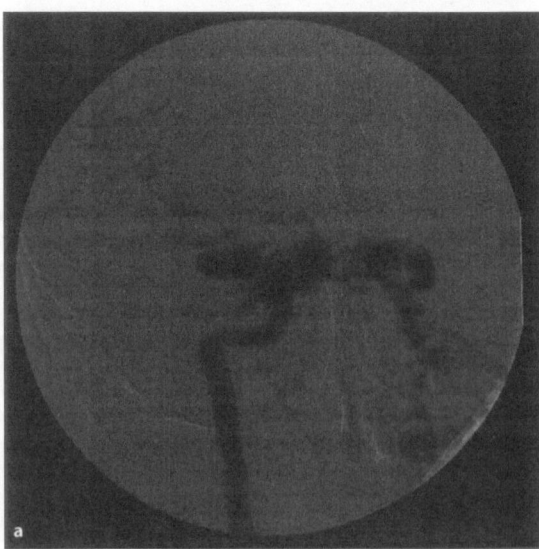

Fig 2. a Right carotid angiography with direct fistula and intracranial hemodynamic effect with no perfusion of A1 and A2.

balloon occlusion if critical stenosis of the internal carotid artery or obliteration of the carrier vessel were to be expected. For a few years now, an alternative to balloon occlusion has existed; it relies on selective embolization of the
fistula by platinum coils within the cavernous sinus. In this case, catheterization can be performed by use of an open-ended catheter with guide wire. This
improves the ability to catheterize even smaller fistulae over the use of balloon
catheters. In addition to this, the handling of coils has improved significantly

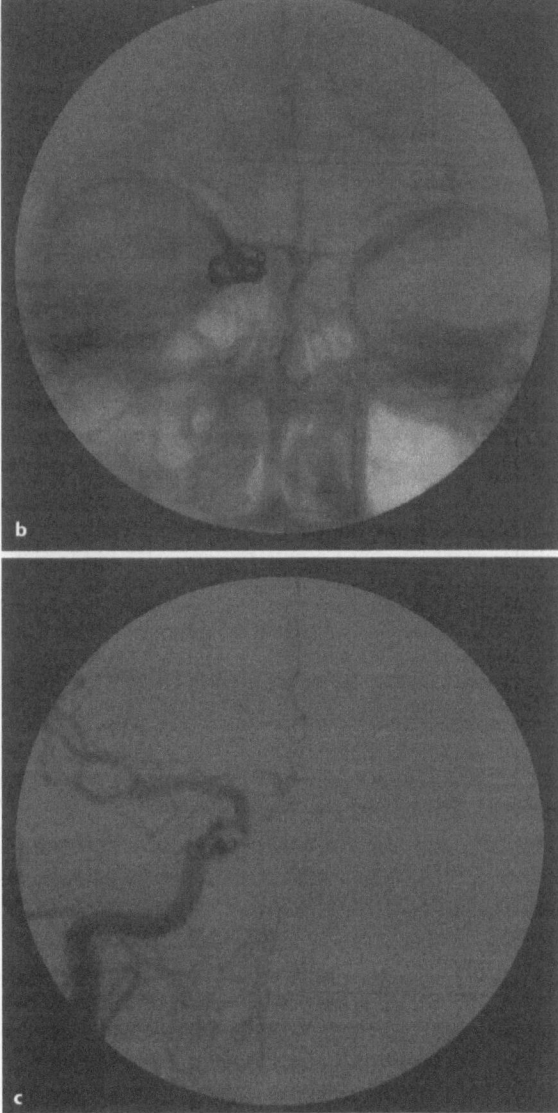

Fig. 2. b Three GDCs in the
fistula. **c** Internal carotid
angiography after endovascular occlusion of the fistula
showing that the fistula is
occluded Immediate hemo-
dynamic effect with perfusion of A1 and A2

since the introduction of Guglielmi detachable coils in the early 1990s [16–18] (Fig. 2a-c).

Another alternative presents the venous approach either via direct puncture/surgical opening of the opthalmic vein or via a transferomal approach with catheterization of the ophthalmic vein and cavernous sinus followed by embolization with platinum coils [4, 19, 21, 25, 27, 30, 31, 33].

References

1. Benati A, Maschio A, Perini S, Beltramello A (1980) Treatment of posttraumatic carotid-cavernous fistula using a detachable balloon catheter. J Neurosurg 53: 784–786
2. Berenstein A, Kricheff I, Ransohoff J (1980) Carotid-cavernous fistulas: intraarterial treatment. Am J Neurol Res 1: 449–457
3. Bitzer M, Bien S (1993) Endovaskuläres Therapiekonzept bei traumatischen Arteria carotis-Sinus cavernosus-Fisteln unter Berücksichtigung neuer Embolisationstechniken. Klin Neuroradiol 3: 63–72
4. Courtheoux P, Labbe D, Hamel C, Lecoq PJ, Jahara M, Théron J (1987) Treatment of bilateral spontaneous dural carotid-cavernous fistulas by coils and sclerotherapy. J Neurosurg 66: 468–470
5. Davie JC, Richardson R (1967) Distal internal carotid thromboembolectomy using a Fogarty catheter in total occlusion. J Neurosurg 22: 171–177
6. Debrun G (1983) Treatment of traumatic carotid-cavernous fistula using detachable balloon catheters. Am J Neurol Res 4: 355–356
7. Debrun G, Lacour P, Caron JP, Hurth M, Comoy J, Keravel Y (1978) Detachable balloon and calibrated-leak balloon techniques in the treatment of cerebral vascular lesions. J Neurosurg 49: 635–649
8. Debrun G, Lacour P, Caron JP, Hurth M, Comoy J, Keravel Y, Loisance D (1975) Traitement de fistules artérioveineuses et d'anéurysmes par ballon gonflable et largable. Nouv Presse Med 4: 2315–2318
9. Debrun G, Lacour P, Caron JP, Hurth M, Comoy J, Keravel Y, Laborit G (1975) Experimental approach of the treatment of carotid-cavernous fistulas with an inflatable and isolated balloon. Neuroradiol 9: 9–12
10. Debrun G, Lacour P, Vinuela F, Fox A, Drake CG, Caron JP (1981) Treatment of 54 traumatic carotid-cavernous fistulas. J Neurosurg 55: 678–692
11. Debrun GM, Vinuela F, Fox AJ, Daves KR, Ahn KS (1988) Indication for treatment of 132 carotid-cavernous fistulas. Neurosurgery 22: 285–289
12. Fierstien SB, DeFeio D, Nutkiewicz A (1978) Complete obliteration of a carotid cavernous fistula with sparing of the carotid blood flow using a detachable balloon catheter. Surg Neurol 9: 277–280
13. Garcia-Cervigon E, Bien S, Laurent A, Weitzner I, Biondi A, Merland JJ (1988) Treatment of a recurrent traumatic carotid-cavernous fistula: vertebro-basilar approach after surgical occlusion of the internal carotid artery. Neuroradiol 30: 355–357
14. Gaston A, Combes C, Razavi F, Le Bras F, Tartiére S, Marsault C (1986) Bilateral posttraumatic carotid-cavernous fistula: anatomico-radiological correlations in a case treated by detachable ballon. J Neuroradiol 13: 55–61
15. Goto K, Hieshima GB, Higashida RT, Halbach VV, Bentson JR, Mehringer CM, Pribram HF (1986) Treatment of direct carotid cavernous sinus fistulae. Acta Radiol Suppl 369: 576–579
16. Guglielmi G, Vinuela F, Sepetka I, Macellari V (1991) Electrothrombosis of saccular aneurysms via endovascular approach. Part 1: electrochemical basis technique and experimental results. J Neurosurg 75: 1–7
17. Guglielmi G, Vinuela F, Dion G, Duckwiler G (1991) Electrothrombosis of saccular aneurysms via endovascular approach. Part 2: preliminary clinical experience. J Neurosurg 75: 8–14

18. Guglielmi G, Vinuela F, Briganti F, Duckwiler G (1992) Carotid-cavernosus fistula caused by a ruptured intracavernous aneurysm: endovascular treatment by electrothrombosis with detachable coils. Neurosurgery 31: 591–597
19. Halbach VV, Higashida RT, Hieshima GB, Hardin CW, Probram H (1989) Transvenous embolization of dural fistulas involving the cavernous sinus. AJNR 10: 377–383
20. Halbach VV, Hieshima GB, Higashida RT, Reicher M (1987) Carotid cavernous fistulae: indications for urgent treatment. Am J Neurol Res 8: 627–633
21. Halbach VV, Higashida RT, Hieshima GB, Hardin CW, Yang PJ (1988) Transvenous embolization of direct carotid cavernous fistulas. Am J Neurol Res 9: 741–747
22. Hamby WB (1966) Carotid cavernous fistula. Thomas, Springfield
23. Helmke K, Laas R, Kühne D (1981) An improved balloon catheter technique for the occlusion of carotid-cavernous sinus fistulas (CCF). Acta Neurochir 59: 87–94
24. Kendall B (1983) Results of treatment of arteriovenous fistulae with the Debrun technique. Am J Neurol Res 4: 405–408
25. Komiyama M, Morikawa K, Fu Y, Yagura H, Yasui T, Baba M (1990) Indirect carotid-cavernous sinus fistula: Transvenous embolization from the external jugular vein using a superior ophthalmic vein approach: a case report. Surg Neurol 33: 57–63
26. Lister JR, Sypert GW (1979) Traumatic false aneurysm and carotid cavernous fistula: a complication of sphenoidotomy. Neurosurgery 5: 473–475
27. Manelfe C, Berenstein A (1 980) Treatment of carotid cavernous fistulas by venous approach. J Neuroradiol 7: 13–21
28. Prolo DJ, Hanberry JW (1971) Intraluminal occlusion of a carotid-cavernous sinus fistula with a balloon catheter: technical note. J Neurosurg 35: 237–242
29. Serbinenko FA (1974) Ballon catheterisation and occlusion of major vessels. J Neurosurg 42: 152–154
30. Shimizu T, Waga S, Kojima T, Tanaka K (1988) Transvenous ballon occlusion of the cavernous sinus: an alternative therapeutic choice for recurrent traumatic carotid-cavernous fistulas. Neurosurgery 22: 550–553
30a.Takahashi U, Kileffer F, Wilson G (1969) Iatrogenic carotid cavernous fistula. J Neurosurg 30: 498–500
31. Teng MH, Guo NY, Huang CI, Wu CC, Chang T (1988) Occlusion of arteriovenous malformations of the cavernous sinus via the superior ophthalmic vein. Am J Neuro Res 9: 539–546
32. Turner DM, VanGilder JC, Mojtahedi S, Dierson EW (1983) Spontaneous intracerebral hematoma in carotid cavernous fistula. J Neurosurg 59: 680–686
33. Uflacker R, Lima S, Ribas GC, Piske R (1986) Carotid-cavernous fistulas: embolization through the superior ophthalmic vein approach. Radiology 159: 175–179

7 Guidelines for the Management of Severe Head Injury: An Overview

R.M. Chesnut

Evidence-Based Guidelines for the Management of Severe Head Injury

Guidelines for the practice of clinical medicine have long been an accepted and useful part of practice. Certainly, in such instances as the management of cardiac tachyarrythmias, status epilepticus, or the initial ABCs of resuscitation, they have lead to optimization of treatment approaches under conditions where time is of the essence. Fortunately, for these topics, there is a great deal of data readily available regarding various treatment methods.

Unfortunately, however, all guidelines are not created equal. Indeed, published guidelines range from empiric, literature-based works to pure expert opinion. Although the utility of practice guidelines does not necessarily parallel their scientific rigor, if controversy is to be avoided and guidelines are to be rapidly accepted and disseminated, it is important that individual recommendations be firmly and explicitly rooted in the available literature. In general, the value of such processes is becoming increasingly well recognized and quite rigorous approaches have been described to assist in the development of practice guidelines [12].

Although guidelines for the management of general trauma under many commonly experienced conditions have been developed and disseminated for many years [1], such is not the case with respect to severe traumatic brain injury (TBI). Indeed, according to a recently published survey, it is entirely possible, and even likely, that a patient suffering a severe TBI [postresuscitation Glasgow Coma Scale (GCS) score $\leq$ 8] who is admitted to a major center that regularly deals with such patients might be managed without an intracranial pressure (ICP) monitor, hyperventilated to a $PaCO_2 < 25$ mm Hg (< 3.3 kPa), given scheduled doses of mannitol, receive barbiturates, be treated with high dose glucocorticoids, and be maintained in an iatrogenic state of systemic volume contraction [13]. The survey upon which such a scenario is founded polled neurotrauma management strategies at 219 trauma centers regularly dealing with severe TBI patients [13]. This survey reported that 43% of such centers monitor ICP less than 50% of the time in patients with severe TBI, with only 28% routinely monitoring ICP monitoring in such patients. Often in the absence of ICP monitoring, osmotic diuretics were used routinely in 83% of centers, steroids were routinely administered in 64% of centers, cerebral spinal fluid drainage was routinely used in 44% of centers, barbiturates were administered in 33% of centers, and 57% of centers routinely hyperventilated to a range of 25–30 mm Hg (3.3–4.0 kPa) with 29% routinely hyperventilating to <25 mm Hg (< 3.3 kPa).

In the practice of clinical medicine, variation in treatment is acceptable, often necessary, and, to some extent, desirable. However, management regimens such as that outlined above represent what appears to be unusual and rather glaring combinations of strategies that are less than widely accepted. Their existence suggests that either there are profound deficits in the literature supporting various methods of managing severe TBI or that there is a serious defect in the dissemination of that which is actually known in this field.

In response to such documented variations in care, a committee of neurosurgeons formed in 1993 to address the scientific literature pertaining to TBI. This committee was composed of ten neurosurgeons whose primary academic interests were clinical and research aspects of severe TBI. The committee was formed in conjunction with the Joint Section on Neurotrauma and Critical Care of the American Association of Neurological Surgeons (AANS) and the Congress of Neurological Surgeons (CNS). It was organized and supported by the Brain Trauma Foundation. Throughout the process involved in developing these guidelines, considerable input and guidance was provided by the Guidelines Committee of the AANS. A large part of their input was focused toward the elaboration and employment of a specific, explicit, literature-based approach to the development of guidelines based on well established protocols [12]. The quality and validity of the Guidelines for the Management of Severe Head Injury are integrally related to their developmental process such that the proper interpretation of the guidelines requires a concomitant understanding of the process itself. Therefore the basics of this approach are outlined below.

Although initially formed by and composed of neurosurgeons, the scope of this effort certainly exceeded this one specific specialty. In addition, because of the global nature of TBI, geographic borders were also artificial. In response to these considerations, input was actively solicited from members of related disciplines as well as international consultants. Throughout the process of the 8+ revisions, input was received from the American College of Surgeons, the American College of Emergency Room Physicians, the American Academy of Neurology, the American College of Physical Medicine and Rehabilitation, and the Society of Critical Care Medicine. In addition, significant input throughout the process was received from neurosurgeons and critical care medicine specialists in the United Kingdom and Europe. Input from international participants was particularly valuable because it broadened the literature base and also was pivotal in avoiding misinterpretations of data arising from perspectives that have become subtly but widely disseminated within the United States.

One of the major goals of the guidelines process was to empirically investigate the quality of existing literature in this field and to determine whether reasonable practice parameters could be developed based entirely on published, peer-reviewed data. As a first step, the following ten topics were selected to be addressed in the first iteration of this effort:

- Trauma systems and the neurosurgeon
- The integration of brain-specific treatment
- Resuscitation of blood pressure and oxygenation
- Indications for ICP monitoring
- ICP treatment threshold
- Recommendations for ICP monitoring technology
- Guidelines for cerebral perfusion pressure
- The use of hyperventilation in acute management
- The use of mannitol in severe head injury
- The use of barbiturates in the control of intracranial hypertension
- The role of glucocorticoids in the treatment of severe head injury
- Critical pathway for the treatment of established intracranial hypertension
- Nutritional support of brain injured patients
- The role of antiseizure prophylaxis following head injury

These topics were felt to be fundamental to the management of severe TBI patients. This list is certainly not exhaustive, and topics such as surgical management, and pediatric issues are added in future iterations. In addition, in keeping with the mandates of the Guidelines Committee of the AANS, the fascicles on each of the present 14 topics are regularly reviewed and revised in light of an increasing literature base.

Each topic was approached in an identical fashion. Once it had been carefully defined, efforts were made to assemble all relevant scientific articles. The one fundamental selection criteria for all publications was that they be focused on human clinical outcome. With that in mind, electronic literature surveys using explicitly defined keyword searches was performed back to 1966. Articles garnered using this approach were supplemented with publications from other sources such as bibliographies, other databases, and generally available albeit not always published results from "negative prospective randomized controlled trials (presented in the section on seizure prophylaxis). All publications so gathered were then reviewed with respect to their experimental design, the methods and success of their clinical execution, and their statistical validity. Using these data, each article was classified using the following three point scale which served to stratify the empiric strength of their conclusions:

- Class I includes only prospective randomized controlled studies that were properly designed, executed, and described.
- Class II includes prospective randomized controlled trials that did not meet the strict criteria for class I as well as nonrandomized prospective controlled trials, large prospectively collected databases, etc.
- Class III includes studies such as case series, case reports, and expert opinion. This classification places the most statistically rigorous investigations into class I and relegates the least controlled reports as well as expert opinion to class III.

The strength of this document is based on the strict linkage between input (stratified, published data) and output (practice parameters). In like manner to the stratification of articles, the practice parameters were classified into three groups depending upon their level of certainty. In descending order, these groups consist of standards, guidelines, and options:

- Standards represent accepted principles of patient management reflecting a high degree of clinical certainty. They are based on class I evidence.
- Guidelines represent a particular strategy or range of management strategies reflecting a moderate clinical certainty. They are based on class II evidence.
- Options reflect patient management strategies for which there is unclear clinical certainty. They are based on class III evidence.

Throughout this process, the classification of individual research articles and their elective incorporation into standards, guidelines, or options was subjected to repeated and vigorous review by the entire committee. The focus and precise wording of each standard, guideline, and option was not finalized until it had been accepted by all members of the committee and input from outside reviewers had been formally considered. The results of each of these steps is explicitly presented in the guidelines document in terms of the classification of articles and their linkage to practice parameters. Those articles felt to be most relevant and upon which the recommendations are most solidly based are presented in evidentiary tables which contain the reference, a summary of the work, the classification of the article, and its contribution to the guidelines process.

The precise linkage between input publications and output statements is the true key to this document. The explicit presentation of the process not only allows the reader to fully understand the development of each statement but also defines the foundation through which any criticisms should be built in that they should follow the same explicit format, either disagreeing with individual analyses of publications or citing publications inadvertently omitted from the analysis. This process formally disallows disagreements with statements at the standards or guidelines levels based on personal experience or expert opinion.

Because of a strong desire by the committee that the entire developmental process be openly linked to the resulting statements, it was decided that a "concise form" of this document would not be developed. The document is only disseminated in toto. In keeping with this policy, the precise standards, guidelines, and options are not presented in the present discussion but rather is abstracted and summarized with respect to their projected impact on TBI management. Since the direct linkage between the publications and practice parameters is so critical and because this linkage is not presented in detail here, references to individual articles during discussion of the guidelines are also avoided here. For the precise wording of the standards, guidelines, and options as well as the process involved in their development, the reader is referred to the guidelines document [4] or the associated formal complete publications in the Journal of Neurotrauma [5] or the European Journal of Emergency Medicine [3]. The original document may be obtained through the Brain Trauma Foundation, 523 E 72nd Street, 8th Floor, New York, NY 10021, USA. Voice (212)772–0608, fax (212)7720357.

Overview

A total of 2941 articles were reviewed during this process. Three hundred forty-two articles were cited in the text. The final product consisted of three standards, ten guidelines, and sixteen options for the fourteen topics.

Trauma Systems

The Guidelines for the Management of Severe Head Injury reflects the evidence in strong support for regionalized trauma systems. The importance of involvement of the neurosurgeon in the development and execution of these systems is emphasized. The critical necessity of having 24 hour capabilities available for rapid clinical diagnosis and management, imaging, emergency surgery, and neurotrauma intensive care management at centers routinely managing severe TBI is supported. In areas where such systems are not available, formal triage protocols must be developed. The routine management of severe TBI patients in the absence of active neurosurgical input or facility availability is improper. In regions where necessary neurosurgical coverage may occasionally be unavailable due to a factor such as geography or weather, the basic surgical procedures required for life saving maneuvers should be known to trauma surgeons at the center.

Initial Resuscitation of the Severe TBI Patient (Injury Through Initiation of ICP Monitoring)

Although there is literature supporting the link between organized emergency medical service delivery and improved outcome from severe TBI, the efficacy of individual management strategies has not been formally investigated. Therefore recommendations in this section had to be based on the several available good studies on the influence of secondary brain insults such as hypotension and hypoxia on outcome [6, 11, 22]. These data were used to formulate the basics of early resuscitation. The guidelines support early and vigorous volume resuscitation of the severe brain injury patient with the goal of establishing systemic blood pressures adequate to support cerebral perfusion. Hypotension [defined in the literature as a systolic blood pressure (SBP) < 90 mm Hg], and hypoxia (defined as apnea or cyanosis in the field or a PaO_2 less than 60 mm Hg) must be avoided whenever possible or immediately corrected when present. There is no support for fluid restriction. Isotonic or hypertonic fluids are recommended. At an option level, an initial goal (prior to insertion of an ICP monitor) of a mean arterial pressure of 90 mm Hg is suggested.

Because of the documented potential hazards of the use of hyperventilation and mannitol and their possible interference with cerebral and systemic resuscitation, their use is not recommended in the general setting of severe TBI unless the patient presents signs of a transtentorial herniation or evidences neurologic deterioration not attributable to extracranial causes. Neither hyperventilation nor mannitol is recommended for "prophylactic" treatment. When there is evidence of intracranial hypertension, however, as manifested by pupillary dilation, motor posturing, or progressive neurologic deterioration not attributable to extracranial causes, the employment of mannitol or hyperventilation is supported. Under such conditions it is expected that critical diagnostic procedures such as CT imaging are expedited.

Indications for ICP Monitoring

There is no literature base for the formulation of ICP monitoring guidelines in patients with moderate (GCS of 9 – 12) or mild (GCS of 13 – 15) traumatic brain injuries. Although it is recognized that monitoring may sometimes be indicated in noncomatose patients, the assessment of indications remains entirely at the discretion of the managing physician.

There is literature support for defining indications for monitoring ICP in severe TBI patients (postresuscitation GCS (8). This literature was reviewed with respect to two basic points: (a) whether the risks of the various methods generally available to lower ICP are sufficiently high that their use should be predicated upon objective measurement of ICP (as opposed to simple "empiric" or "prophylactic" employment); and (b) whether the monitoring of ICP in the management of intracranial hypertension is associated with improved outcome. Analysis of data relevant to the first issue found notable risks associated with such use of hyperventilation, mannitol, neuromuscular blockade, and barbiturates to the extent that their use in severe TBI patients with a well-defined high probability of intracranial hypertension, in the absence of documentation of that hypertension, is not supported. This is especially true for hyperventilation, where the data suggests significant risks, particularly during the acute postinjury period, so that the use of hyperventilation in patients without intracranial hypertension should be strictly avoided.

Concerning the issue of the relationship between the management of intracranial hypertension and improved outcome, there is an unfortunate lack of class I evidence in this regard. Much of the lack of class I evidence regarding this issue is rooted in ethical issues. These arose because ICP monitoring became a well-accepted part of neurotrauma practice in the 1970s based on class II and class III data to the extent that ethical considerations voiced by reviewing groups have prevented funding of subsequent class I studies due to issues regarding control groups. As a result of the lack of prospective randomized controlled trials in this area we will probably always be relegated to the use of class II data. In this light, the most powerful contributing study is that of Eisenberg et al. [9]. Although this was a prospective randomized controlled trial of barbiturates versus the continuation of conventional medical treatment without barbiturates, the final clinical outcome variable measured in this study was control of ICP and not patient outcome. Therefore the analysis of this study with respect to patient outcome relegates it to the class II level. Nevertheless, this study presents rather convincing evidence that the control of intracranial hypertension in patients previously refractory to "conventional medical ICP lowering therapy" was strongly statistically associated with improved outcome regardless of the method through which ICP control was attained. This is powerful evidence that the control of intracranial hypertension is associated with improved outcome.

The above considerations, therefore, support the use of ICP monitoring to direct the management of patients with a reasonable probability of actually having intracranial hypertension. This patient population has been defined [19]. There are two distinct groups with risks of intracranial hypertension of over 60%. The first of these is severe TBI (GCS (8) patients with abnormal CT scans. These CT abnormalities are defined as fractures, contusions, hematomas, midline shift, or compression of the basal cisterns. The second group is patients with severe TBI with normal CT scans who have two or three of the following factors:

- Age greater than 40 years
- Unilateral or bilateral motor posturing
- An episode of systolic blood pressure less than 90 mmHg.

Based on these considerations, the Guidelines for the Management of Severe Head Injury state, at a guidelines level, that severe TBI patients falling into these two groups should receive ICP monitoring.

Recommendations for ICP Monitoring Technology

Given the critical role of ICP monitoring in the management of severe TBI, it was felt desirable to review the available technology. Since technology review is not amenable to outcome based analysis, this is the one section of the Guidelines for the Management of Severe Head Injury that did not produce standards, guidelines, or options. Instead, it produced a set of recommendations.

By virtue of precedence, fluid coupled monitoring of ICP through a ventricular catheter has become the reference standard. In terms of monitoring accuracy, fluid coupled, fiberoptic, or strain-gauge devices placed in the ventricle or brain parenchyma are comparable. Subarachnoid, subdural, or epidural monitors do not provide comparable accuracy and are not recommended as equivalent substitutes. Ventricular catheters have the added utility of allowing therapeutic CSF drainage.

The data regarding complications is somewhat unclear. The precise definition of device-related infection and its differentiation from colonization has not been adequately determined. This is relevant because device-related colonization may be treated simply by removal of the device since it does not represent true infection. Within the limits of difficulties imposed by the lack of definition, it appears that the incidence of infectious complications appears to vary little between devices. Similarly, the incidence of insertion related hemorrhage in patients without coagulopathies appears to be low.

ICP Treatment Threshold

In like manner to the situation for indications for ICP monitoring, the passive integration of 20–25 mm Hg into ICP management strategies that occurred pari passu with the development of ICP management has prevented prospective empiric studies of ICP thresholds in human patients. Although a number of studies have been done correlating outcome with treatment thresholds in a narrow range, as well as comparing observed ICP values with survival, there is an inherent confounding in such analyses because ICP treatment thresholds were always a part of the management strategies. Despite this confounding, however, there is a good deal of class II evidence, incorporating controls for other predictive or confounding variables, suggesting that the operational definition of intracranial hypertension should generally be set at 20–25 mm Hg, at least as the initial value. It is noted, however, that the use of any treatment threshold should be correlated with the clinical examination and the cerebral perfusion pressure.

Management of Cerebral Perfusion Pressure

Despite the Sturm und Drang surrounding cerebral perfusion pressure management, its firm establishment as a scientific principle remains impeded by the absence of prospectively collected, parallel control groups in the literature. Therefore the supporting literature remains at the class III level. Nevertheless, there is a number of highly suggestive class III studies which are well supported by firm physiology. The Guidelines for the Management of Severe Head Injury recommends, at an option level, that cerebral perfusion pressure should be maintained (70 mm Hg throughout the acute care course of the severe TBI patient. During resuscitation, prior to the time of insertion of an ICP monitor, when cerebral perfusion pressure cannot be calculated, it is recommended (also at an option level) that the target mean arterial pressure be 90 mm Hg.

The Use of Mannitol in Severe TBI

Although its efficacy has never been studied independently of other factors, the use of mannitol is supported in the management of intracranial hypertension. It is recognized that this use must be predicated upon the avoidance of systemic volume contraction due to the induced diuresis as well as serum hyperosmolarity. Doses of 0.25 g/kg appear equally effective in lowering ICP as doses of 1.0 g/kg. Mannitol is more effective when administered in bolus form than as a continuous infusion.

The Use of Hyperventilation in the Acute Management of Severe TBI

Hyperventilation is one area in which a standard could be developed. Unfortunately, this is based on a single class I study [18] and, therefore, the wording of the standard quite specifically reflects the design and results of that study. At a standard level, it is stated that chronic, prolonged hyperventilation therapy at a $PaCO_2 \leq 25$ mm Hg (≤ 3.3 kPa) should not be used in the absence of increased ICP after severe TBI. At the class II (guidelines) level, there are more supportive studies and the breadth of the statement can be increased. The guideline for hyperventilation states that the use of prophylactic hyperventilation of any degree [$PaCO_2 < 35$ mm Hg (< 4.6 kPa)] should be avoided during the first 24 h after severe TBI.

Based on the standard and the guideline, the use of prophylactic hyperventilation is not supported in TBI. This is consistent with the recommendations for the prehospital period when ICP monitoring is not available and hyperventilation is suggested to be used only when there are clinical signs of increased ICP. In addition, since the use of hyperventilation for prophylaxis is not supported, it directly supports the insertion of an ICP monitor in any patient with a TBI felt severe enough to be at risk for intracranial hypertension. The employment of hyperventilation as a treatment for severe TBI in patients without ICP monitors is not supported.

Hyperventilation therapy may be necessary under two conditions. It may be used for brief periods when there is acute neurologic deterioration (such as during the prehospital period or in the Intensive Care Unit during spikes of ICP that need to be rapidly reduced). Under such conditions there is concomitant activation of mechanisms to diagnose and treat the underlying causes of this episode. Secondly, hyperventilation therapy may be necessary for longer periods if there is intracranial hypertension that is refractory to therapeutic maneuvers with more favorable risk: benefit ratios (e. g., sedation, neuromuscular blockade, CSF drainage, osmotic diuretics, and cerebral perfusion pressure management).

The Use of Barbiturates in the Control of Intracranial Hypertension

Of the various treatments for intracranial hypertension, barbiturates has been subjected to the greatest number of prospective randomized controlled trials. Such investigations have promoted the realization the barbiturates are not effective as prophylaxis against intracranial hypertension [26] or as a substitute for mannitol in the early treatment of intracranial hypertension in nonselected patients [24]. As noted previously, the study by Eisenberg et al. did show that barbiturates were quite effective in lowering ICP that had previously been refractory to other methods of medical management [9]. As discussed in the section on indications for ICP monitoring, because the Eisenberg study used ICP control and not patient outcome as its primary dependent variable, this study is actually class II with respect to outcomes although class I with respect to ICP control. Therefore the statement regarding barbiturates is made at the guidelines level. This statement supports the consideration of the use of barbiturates in patients with intracranial hypertension that is refractory to methods with a more favorable risk: benefit ration [e.g., sedation, neuromuscular blockade, cerebral perfusion pressure therapy, CSF drainage, mannitol, and hyperventilation to 30 – 35 mm Hg (4.0 – 4.6 kPa)]. Within the judgment of the managing physician, such patients should be felt to be "salvageable" in that the primary ongoing problem is not the severity of the initial injury but rather ongoing secondary insults. Candidate patients should also be experiencing problems with hypotension prior to barbiturate administration. This guideline does not mandate that barbiturates be used in such patients but merely that they should be considered when ICP proves refractory to the extent that "second tier" therapies are considered.

Critical Pathway for the Treatment of Established Intracranial Hypertension

Over the 3 year process of reviewing the almost 5000 articles involved in this project, a general sense arose of what appeared to be a treatment approach that is most consistent with the body of published evidence. Although there has been little investigation of the interactions between various treatment modalities, an understanding of their efficacy along with their risk: benefit ratios allows the formulation of a treatment algorithm albeit only at an expert opinion (option) level. The critical pathway that is contained in the Guidelines for the Management of Severe Head Injury represents such a class III algorithm which, although founded on a concomitant and in-depth analysis of an exhaustive collection of the literature, remains a consensus opinion. Nevertheless, it should be useful in the formulation of a basic strategy for managing TBI patients. Certainly, however, as a class III algorithm, it is expected that it be readily modified in its application to individual patients at the discretion of the managing physician.

The algorithm is divided into two sections, hinging upon the insertion of an ICP monitor. The first session starts at initial patient contact and fundamentally invokes full resuscitation of the patient (Fig. 1). The initial resuscitation revolves around the ABC's of the Advanced Trauma Life Support (ATLS) protocols [1]. The goal is complete physiologic resuscitation to euvolemia, with strict avoidance of hypotension (systolic blood pressure < 90 mm Hg) and a suggested mean arterial pressure goal of 90 mm Hg. Prevention of hypoxia, maintenance of ventilation, and airway protection are also critical and often mandate endotracheal intubation and assisted ventilation. Under no conditions are these patients treated with fluid restriction.

Since these patients are often uncooperative, and since even apparently comatose patients respond physiologically to noxious stimulation, the use of

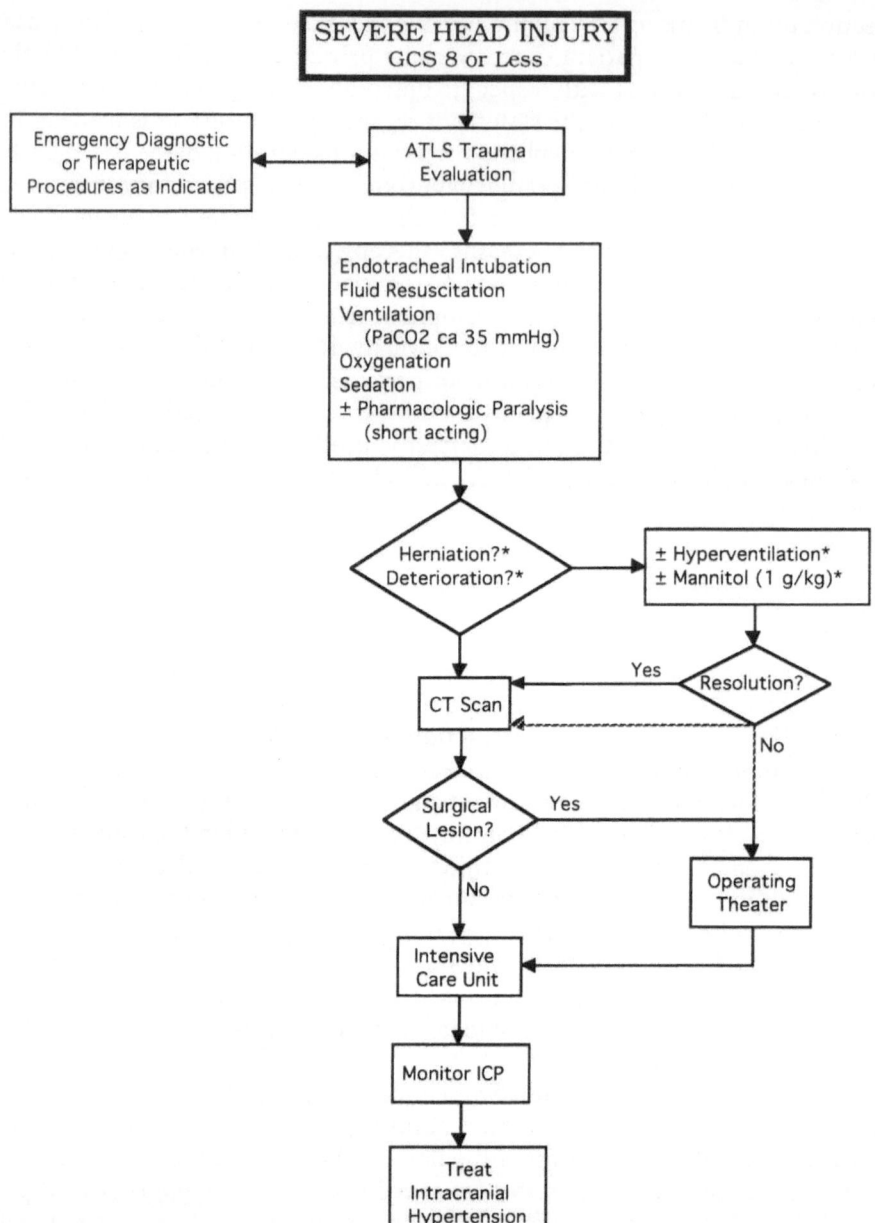

Fig. 1. Initial resuscitation of the severely head-injured patient (treatment options).
* Only in the presence of signs of herniation or progressive neurological deterioration not attributable to extracranial factors

sedation and analgesia is well supported. Neuromuscular blockade may be administered for purposes of transport, keeping in mind that it does eliminate the neurologic examination. Hyperventilation or mannitol is employed only in the presence of evidence of increased ICP as manifest by motor or pupillary changes or progressive neurologic deterioration not attributable to other causes.

TBI patients are rapidly transported to a trauma center with appropriate and available neurosurgical coverage. The resuscitation is continued and completed there intercurrent to emergent CT imaging of the brain and stabilization of life-threatening extracranial injuries. Pending other emergent diagnostic or therapeutic maneuvers, the patient may go to the operating theater or directly to the Intensive Care Unit. Upon arrival in the Intensive Care Unit the goal is the attainment and maintenance of normal homeostatic physiology in all systems supplemented by supporting the mean arterial pressure at 90 mm Hg. At the earliest possible point during the resuscitation, an ICP monitor is inserted and therapy thereafter directed toward lowering ICP and maintaining cerebral perfusion pressure at 70 mm Hg or more.

The second algorithm begins upon the insertion of an ICP monitor (Fig. 2). Irrespective of the presence or absence of intracranial hypertension, the initial goal is the maintenance of a cerebral perfusion pressure of 70 mm Hg. When intracranial hypertension obtains, the first treatment is CSF drainage when ventricular access is available. In some cases, this may be all that is needed to control ICP. It should be remembered that the ICP cannot be accurately measured if the catheter is open to drainage. Therefore measurements must be obtained with the drainage system closed.

If CSF drainage is not adequate to control intracranial hypertension, the agent with next most favorable risk: benefit ratio appears to be mannitol. Mannitol should be administered in conjunction with the recommendations discussed above. If mannitol is not effective or further administration is prevented due to problems with volume contraction or hyperosmolarity, hyperventilation may be employed to 30 – 35 mm Hg. This would be the first point at which iatrogenic hypocapnia would be employed.

In the instance where this degree of hyperventilation is not effective, one enters the realm of "second tier therapy." This level of treatment should be recognized as "uncharted waters." The best studied of these second tier therapies is the use of high dose barbiturates. As noted previously, there is no class I evidence supporting the efficacy of high dose barbiturates in improving outcome and there are no studies at all comparing it to other second tier therapies. With respect to other treatment methods, there is a wide variation in the number and quality of supporting studies. At the first iteration of the Guidelines for the Management of Severe Head Injury, none of them has as yet been covered as a topic. Therefore no statement is made with respect to the process through which the selection of a second tier therapy in the management of a given patient should be accomplished. Given the quality of available research, it is reasonable that barbiturates be considered but this certainly does not

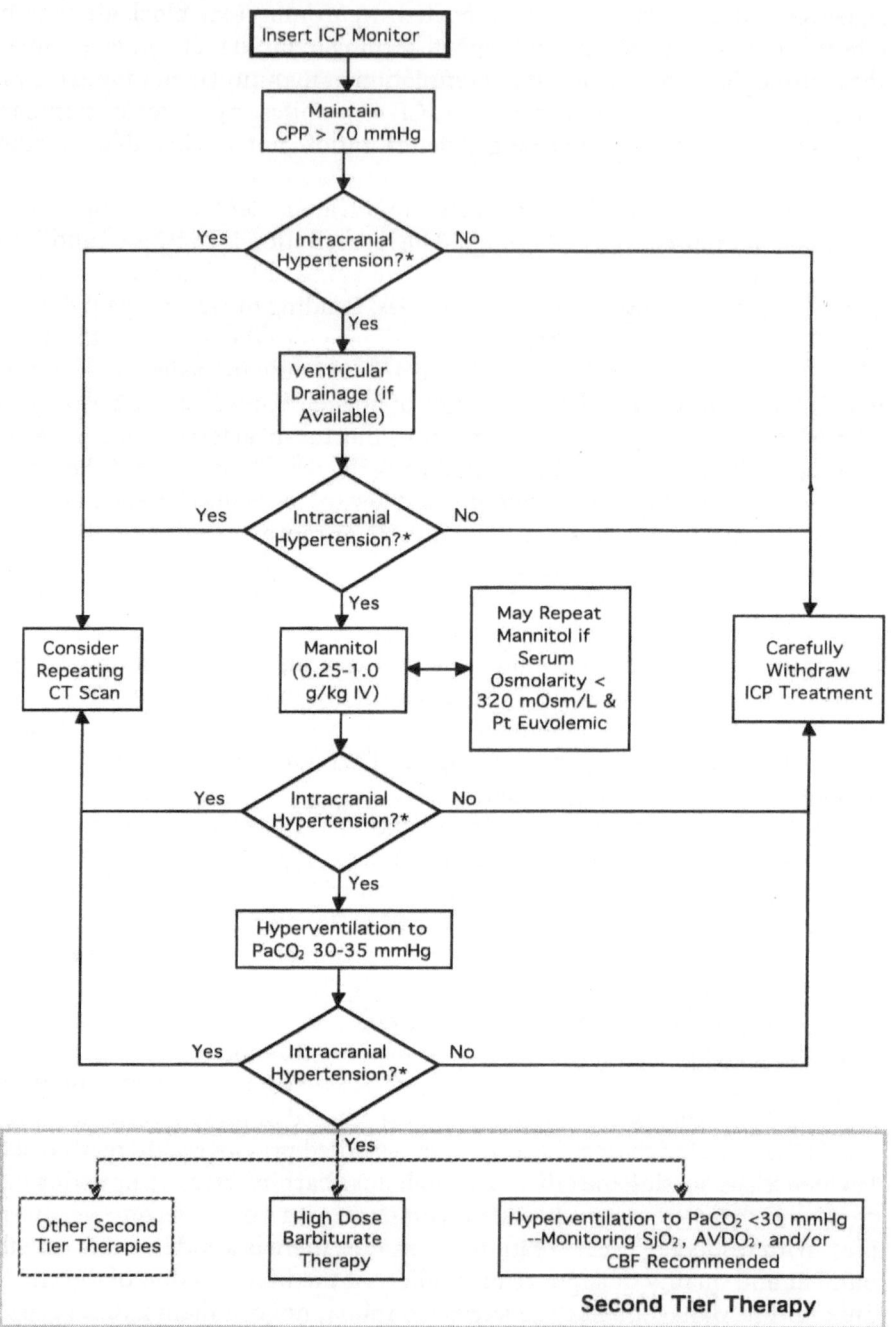

Fig. 2. Critical pathway for treatment of intracranial hypertension in the severely head-injured patient (treatment options).
* Threshold of 20–25 mm Hg may be used; other values may be substituted in individual conditions

imply that they be used. Future iterations of the Guidelines for the Management of Severe Head Injury will deal with alternative second tier therapies.

At all points during the treatment of intracranial hypertension, the possibility of a surgical cause of the elevated ICP should be entertained. When such a possibility cannot be clinically eliminated, consideration should be given to repeated CT imaging.

Use of Glucocorticoids in the Management of Severe TBI

Based on six class I reports, none of which found statistically significant improvement in ICP or outcome in the inception cohort of severe TBI patients, the Guidelines for the Management of Severe Head Injury make a standard level statement that the use of glucocorticoids is not supported for the control of ICP or the improvement of outcome in patients with severe TBI [2, 7, 8, 10, 14, 23]. Notably, this is not in accord with common practice, as demonstrated in the survey of TBI management strategies by Ghajar et al. [13]. In the light of available, peer-reviewed literature, however, it would appear that the alteration of such practice is in order.

Seizure Prophylaxis in TBI

Consistent with the approach taken in the literature, the analysis of available evidence on seizure prophylaxis was interpreted in terms of short-term and long-term efficacy. Short-term is defined as the first two weeks following trauma with long-term commencing thereafter. There are seven class I studies dealing with the use of antiseizure prophylaxis following severe TBI [15 – 17, 20, 21, 25, 27]. These studies do not support the use of phenytoin, carbamazepine, or phenobarbital as being statistically effective in preventing the development of late posttraumatic seizures. It is to be noted that these investigations were not primarily outcome studies. Nevertheless, since such treatments were not effective in diminishing the incidence of such seizures, the absence of a beneficial influence on outcome is a proper inference.

With respect to the short-term, the situation is somewhat different. There is class I evidence that early management does decrease the incidence of seizures during the acute course. There is, however, no evidence that this diminution is associated with improved outcome. In conjunction with the known side effects of anticonvulsant medications, some of which are serious, the absence of data directly addressing the correlation of a decreased incidence of acute seizures with improved outcome severely confounds the interpretation of this data. Therefore the choice of employing anticonvulsant medications for the prophylaxis of acute posttraumatic seizures is left to the discretion of the physician. If it is felt important to manage acute posttraumatic seizures prophylactically, anticonvulsant administration may be chosen. If it is felt that the risks outweigh the benefits, there is also justification for not administering such medications. When making such decisions, less well studied factors such as the ability or lack thereof to detect seizures should they occur as well as the possible influence of seizure activity on ongoing treatment efforts should be considered.

Nutritional Support of Brain Injured Patients

There is class II evidence supporting the efficacy of early nutrition in decreasing the systemic complications associated with increased morbidity and mortality in TBI patients. Goals are 140 % of basic metabolic requirements in patients not receiving neuromuscular blockade and 100 % of basic metabolic requirements in patients who are pharmacologically relaxed. The enteral route of feeding is preferred.

Implications for Clinical Practice

This edition of the Guidelines for the Management of Severe Head Injury represents the first iteration of an active, "living" process. Due to the evolutionary nature of ongoing research, none of the statements made in this document should be interpreted as immutable. It is anticipated, indeed desired, that future research either increase the class of support for such statements or refute them based on improved experimental design or execution. In addition, these fourteen topics certainly do not cover the gamut of neurotrauma issues. Extremely important topics such as pediatric issues, surgical management, etc. are not covered. It is intended that the next iteration not only include updated versions of the present fascicles but also new topics.

The rigorous and explicit nature of the process through which these guidelines were developed should make them author independent. Certainly, at the levels of standards and guidelines, a concerted effort has been made to exclude personal or expert opinion. However, given the vagaries existent in any individual care setting, the processes involved in the integration of these guidelines into clinical practice must be made on a site- or patient-specific basis. Such implementation may require significant effort and perforce involves emergency medical services personnel, emergency department personnel, trauma surgeons, critical care surgeons, and anesthesiologists, as well as neurosurgeons, to ensure consistency and continuity of care. Although the Guidelines for the Management of Severe Head Injury may be seen as providing some of the building blocks, the development of delivery systems germane to specific applications obviously involves a great deal of local effort.

Since they are based on class I evidence, the integration of standards into clinical practice should be fairly straightforward. As such, it is anticipated that standards will soon become the standards of care. It is notable, however, that standards should not be interpreted as standards of care in a legal sense unless and until they have become incorporated into the management routines employed by a significant fraction of physicians practicing in a given community.

Based on class II evidence guidelines are better supported than their available alternatives. Therefore it is anticipated that they will also be eventually incorporated into standards of practice. An important caveat with respect to this process, however, is that the class II level of support of guidelines-level statements needs to be kept in mind and that such statements should be subjected to class I investigations for the purpose of further proof or refutation whenever possible.

With respect to treatment options, the course of their integration into standards of practice is undefined. Because their superiority over alternate treatment methods is unclear by definition, the propriety of their application in a given instance remains entirely at the discretion of the physician. In many cases the impression of their general preferability over other approaches may be obviated by immediate ancillary considerations. In general, the recommendations contained in option-level statements should be considered under applicable circumstances without any specific implications with respect to their application.

The Guidelines for the Management of Severe Head Injury serve as an empiric synopsis of existing literature on fourteen topics relevant to the management of severe TBI patients. As such, they should not be seen as a mandate but, rather, as a literature resource for those involved in this aspect of medicine. Intended to facilitate the development of evidence-based management protocols, they necessarily address all of the related disciplines involved in TBI care. As such, they should greatly facilitate the development of management strategies that can be shared amongst a wide variety of centers, therefore obviating the inconsistencies documented by the survey of Ghajar et al. [13].

With respect to the numerous aspects of TBI management not covered in this document, the strategies are left entirely to the discretion of the physician with the somewhat onerous corollary that they should be based as much as possible on empiric analysis of peer-reviewed literature. In instances where this is straightforward, the outcome should not be effected. In instances where care is unusually complex or the literature is unclear, however, these limitations should be formally recognized and the possible utility of expert consultation or referral of patients to specialty centers be considered. Such referrals should serve not only to improve the care of selected patients by capitalizing on the availability of limited or specialized resources but should also facilitate quality research into controversial or unclear areas by centers with such specific interests.

It is often as important to recognize what we do not know as what we do know. In addition, when there is data on a topic, it is critical that we recognize the quality of evidence supporting given positions. As clearly evidenced in the Guidelines for the Management of Severe Head Injury, the publication of a given study often is more reflective of its relative than its absolute quality. In light of the difficulties as well as the sheer amount of effort involved in the development of evidence-based practice guidelines, it is hoped that the Guidelines for the Management of Severe Head Injury will be a useful tool in its present iteration as well as in the future.

References

1. American College of Surgeons Committee on Trauma (1985) advanced trauma life support course for physicians, instructor manual, 2nd edn. American College of Surgeons, pp 1–525
2. Braakman R, Schouten HJ, Blaauw-van Dishoeck M, Minderhoud JM (1983) Megadose steroids in severe head injury. Results of a prospective double-blind clinical trial. J Neurosurg 58(3): 326–330
3. Bullock R, Chesnut R, Clifton G et al (1996) Guidelines for the management of severe head injury. Eur J Emerg Med 3(2): 109-1-27
4. Bullock R, Chesnut R, Clifton G et al (1996) Guidelines for the management of severe head injury. Brain Trauma Foundation, New York
5. Bullock R, Chesnut R, Clifton G et al (1996) Guidelines for the management of severe head injury. J Neurotrauma 13(11): 639–734
6. Chesnut RM, Marshall LF, Klauber MR et al (1993) The role of secondary brain injury in determining outcome from severe head injury. J Trauma 34(2): 216–222
7. Cooper P, Moody S, Clark W et al (1979) Dexamethasone and severe head injury. A prospective double blind study. J Neurosurg 51: 307–316
8. Dearden NM, Gibson JS, McDowall DG, Gibson RM, Cameron MM (1986) Effect of high-dose dexamethasone on outcome from severe head injury. J Neurosurg 64 (1): 81–88
9. Eisenberg HM, Frankowski RF, Contant CF, Marshall LF, Walker MD (1988) High-dose barbiturate control of elevated intracranial pressure in patients with severe head injury. J Neurosurg 69(1): 15–23
10. Faupel G, Reulen HJ, Muller D (1976) Double-blind study on the effects of steroids on severe closed head injury. In: Pappius HM, Feindel W (ed) Dynamics of brain edema. Springer, Berlin Heidelberg New York, pp 337–343
11. Fearnside MR, Cook RJ, McDougall P, McNeil RJ (1993) The Westmead Head Injury Project outcome in severe head injury. A comparative analysis of pre-hospital, clinical and CT variables. Br J Neurosurg 7(3): 267–279
12. Field MJ, Lohr KN (1992) Guidelines for clinical practice, from development to use. National Acadamy Press, Washington
13. Ghajar J, Hariri RJ, Narayan RK, Iacono LA, Firlik K, Patterson RH (1995) Survey of critical care management of comatose, head-injured patients in the United States. Crit Care Med 3: 560–567
14. Giannotta SL, Weiss MH, Apuzzo ML, Martin E (1984) High dose glucocorticoids in the management of severe head injury. Neurosurgery 15 (4): 497–501
15. Glotzner FL, Haubitz I, Miltner F, Kapp G, Pflughaupt KW (1983) Anfallsprophylaze mit carbamazepin nach schweren schadelhirnverletzungen. Neurochirurgia 26(3): 66–79
16. Manaka S (1992) Cooperative prospective study on posttraumatic epilepsy: risk factors and the effect of prophylactic anticonvulsant. Jpn J Psychiatry Neurology 46(2): 311–315·
17. McQueen JK, Blackwood DH, Harris P, Kalbag RM, Johnson AL (1983) Low risk of late post-traumatic seizures following severe head injury: implications for clinical trials of prophylaxis. J Neurol Neurosurg Psychiatry 46(10): 899–904
18. Muizelaar JP, Marmarou A, Ward JD et al (1991) Adverse effects of prolonged hyperventilation in patients with severe head injury: a randomized clinical trial. J Neurosurg 75(5): 731–739
19. Narayan RK, Kishore PR, Becker DP et al (1982) Intracranial pressure: to monitor or not to monitor? A review of our experience with severe head injury. J Neurosurg 56(5): 650–659
20. Pechadre JC, Lauxerois M, Colnet G et al (1991) Prevention de l'epelepsie post-traumatique tardive par phenytoine dans les traumatismes carniens graves: suivi durant 2 ans. Presse Med Paris 20(18): 841–845

21. Penry JK, White BG, Brackett CE (1979) A controlled prospective study of the pharmacologic prophylaxis of posttraumatic epilepsy. Neurology 29: 600a
22. Pigula FA, Wald SL, Shackford SR, Vane DW (1993) The effect of hypotension and hypoxia on children with severe head injuries. J Pediatr Surg 28(3): 310–314 (discussion 315–316)
23. Saul T, Ducker T, Saleman M, Carro E (1981) Steroids in severe head injury. A prospective, randomized clinical trial. J Neurosurg 54: 596–600
24. Schwartz ML, Tator CH, Rowed DW, Reid SR, Meguro K, Andrews DF (1984) The University of Toronto head injury treatment study: a prospective, randomized comparison of pentobarbital and mannitol. Can J Neurol Sci 11(4): 434–140
25. Temkin NR, Dikmen SS, Winn HR (1991) Management of head injury. Posttraumatic seizures (review). Neurosurg Clin North Am 2(2): 425–135
26. Ward JD, Becker DP, Miller JD et al (1985) Failure of prophylactic barbiturate coma in the treatment of severe head injury. J Neurosurg 62(3): 383–388
27. Young B, Rapp RP, Norton JA, Haack D, Tibbs PA, Bean JR (1983) Failure of prophylactically administered phenytoin to prevent late posttraumatic seizures. J Neurosurg 58(2): 236–241

8 Cranial Fractures and Traumatic Hematomas

R. Firsching

Introduction

The management of fractures and traumatic hematomas is at the core of surgery in neurotraumatology. Often only a few minutes make the difference between recovery and catastrophy. Thus swift and targeted management is of crucial importance. The pathology, diagnosis, and operative measures are outlined below for fractures and hematomas. In real life, however, multiple injuries of course often occur together.

Fractures

Pathology

Fractures result from the degree, location, and direction of energy absorbed. Three morphological types of fractures may be distinguished:

- Linear fracture: fissure of variable width without isolated bone fragments or bone displacement
- Depressed fracture: dislocation of one or multiple fragments usually intracranially, possibly also extracranially
- Comminuted fractures: multiple fragments, often with severe deformity of the skull

It has proven convenient to differentiate fractures according to their location, into fractures of the base of the skull and fractures of the vault [3], as their respective treatments differ. Differentiation of closed and compound fractures of the vault is essential, as compound fractures require operative treatment to reduce the risk of infection. The complications of practical and prognostic relevance associated with skull fractures are lesions of the underlying tissue.

Major complications are intracranial hematomas and cerebrospinal fluid (CSF) fistulas. A probability of 25 % has been reported for a surgically relevant intracranial hematoma with disturbed consciousness in the presence of a skull fracture [29]. By contrast, in oriented patients without a skull fracture the likelihood of an intracranial hematoma is as low as 1 in 6000. Jennett and Teasdale [25] found fractures associated with intracranial hematomas in about 10 % of patients, but 90 % of allepidural hematomas were associated with a skull fracture. Skull fractures in combination with coma grade and mass lesions have been reported to be of predictive value [36].

Diagnosis

Plain skull X-ray has frequently been claimed to disclose a skull fracture. Special projections are necessary for fractures of the posterior fossa. With increasingly sophisticated computed tomography (CT) skull X-ray is no longer indicated [13], and CT has practically replaced conventional tomography. For concomitant CSF leaks several contrast medium investigations were used in the past, namely isotopes and CT cisternography [15]. Magnetic resonance imaging (MRI) has replaced these, as water is displayed with sharp contrast on T2-weighted images.

Operative Measures

Fractures of the vault in which depression exceeds the thickness of the adjacent skull bone are usually associated with a lesion of the dura [20]. This is reason enough for many surgeons to elevate the depression [20] and repair the fractured bone with the use of sutures or miniplates or to replace the bone with methylacrylate cement or other materials. Favorable results in depressed fractures have also been reported after a conservative approach, provided the patients are fully conscious and without significant neurological deficits [5].

Fractures of the base of the skull usually do not require surgery because of a mass effect but because of concomitant CSF leak. All most all cases of petrous bone fractures with CSF otorrhea heal spontaneously within 3 weeks [20]. Treatment of CSF rhinorrhea following a frontobasal fracture is treated in various ways. When the fistula closes spontaneously after several days of CSF drainage, sealing of the leak may be verified by MRI on T2-weighted images. A persistent leak after fracture of the frontal base must be repaired to achieve protection from early or delayed meningitis. There is no consensus on the approach. An extracranial approach may be successful in some cases, but neurosurgeons usually have more confidence in an intracranial intra- or extradural approach.

The timing of surgery of fractures is also controversial. Early surgical débridement has been reported to reduce infection rate significantly [28]. In depressed fractures of the vault causing mass effect early decompression is warranted in the hope of reversing neurological deficits. A conservative approach may be considered in depressed fractures crossing a major venous sinus. The timing of CSF fistula repair is of critical importance as posttraumatic swelling and edema of the brain may complicate surgery. Early repair for fear of infection is not justified as the infection rate during the first 3 weeks is as low as 3% [27] and is not lowered with early repair. Therefore repair of the dura should be delayed until a nearly normal ICP is reached, and the general condition of the patient is stable. A comparative study has shown that this delay of nonvital surgery until the patient is fit results in a marked reduction in mortality [27].

Decompression of the optic nerve has been a matter of controversy for years. The function of the optic nerve may be difficult to assess in the comatose patient. Visual evoked potentials may be helpful in identifying a lesion of the optic nerve [12].

Traumatic Hematomas

Pathology

Epidural Hematomas

Epidural hematomas (synonyms: extradural and peridural hematomas) are collections of blood between dura and skull bone caused by torn dural vessels or oozing from broken skull bone. The high coincidence of epidural hematomas with skull fractures has been outlined above. An interval free of clinical signs of variable duration is sometimes observed.

The course of epidural hematomas over time is therefore of great clinical relevance. Few data are available on the size and volume of epidural hematomas within 1 h of the headinjury, principally because it usually takes more than 1 h until the initial CT is performed. The volumes found within 1 h of the injury clearly do cause a mass effect (see Fig. 1) [17]. In the second and later hours after the injury epidural hematomas can clearly cause a mass effect, making immediate evacuation a life-saving procedure. Mortality clearly increases with the size of the hematoma (see Fig. 2). These may occur at any age but are more frequent in adolescents and young adults. Infrequently they are disclosed by CT after more than 1 day. As recovery of the brain depends on the degree and duration of pressure exerted by the hematoma, the timing of diagnosis is of crucial importance. If it takes about 1 h for the hematoma to accumulate to cause a mass effect, leaving no more than 1 h for acute life-saving measures such as resuscitation, ventilation, treatment of shock, adequate sedation, and transportation.

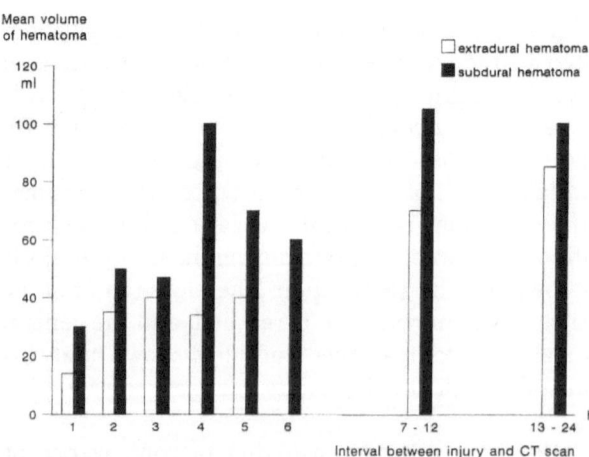

Fig. 1. Relationship of volumes of epidural and subdural hematomas to the length of time between injury and initial CT. Data from 42 epidural and 102 acute subdural hematomas

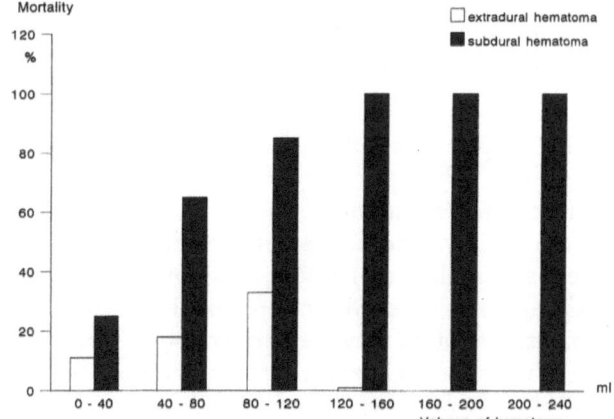

Fig. 2. Relationship of volume of hematomas with mortality. Subdural hematomas beyond a volume of 120 cm³ obviously did not survived

Overall mortality from epidural hematomas is less than 20 % [1, 24]. The urgency of early operation of epidural hematoma is obvious; mortality has been reported to be 32 % in the 2nd hour and 43 % in the 3rd [19]. For patients operated on within 6 h of the injury overall mortality is reported to be 35 % [26]. Concomitant clinical signs such as pupillary responses, motor responses, size of hematomas [17], and associated brain lesions obviously have a bearing on the prognosis. By contrast, patients operated on after more than 12 h have a mortality of 0 % [19].

Subdural Hematomas
Subdural hematomas are collections of blood in the subdural space. The blood usually accumulates either from bridging veins or from lacerations of brain tissue. They are encountered at any interval after the injury, immediately after the injury or even months later. The characteristic feature of subdural hematomas is their high mortality from early hematomas; this has been reported in acute subdural hematomas to be generally higher than 50 % [10]. Becker et al. [2] found a mortality ranging from 57 % to 90 %. Mortality of hematomas identified in the first hour after the head injury has a mortality of 88 % [19]. In hematomas identified in the second hour it decreases to 62 % and in those identified in the third hour to 58 %. From the 2nd to 10th days mortality decreases further, to less than 20 %. After the 10th day the formation of membranes enclosing the hematoma is observed either macroscopically or histologically [6, 16, 21].

An increasing volume of acute subdural hematomas may be distinguished in the first 5 h after the injury (see Fig. 1). Mortality clearly depends on the volume. No acute subdural hematoma larger than 200 cm3 has been survived in our experience (see Fig. 2). From these findings an arbitrary temporal classification of subdural hematomas similar to that suggested by others [21, 32, 34, 35] seems appropriate:

- Acute: symptoms within 24 h of injury
- Subacute: symptoms within 2–10 days
- Chronic: symptoms after the 10th day

Other temporal classifications have also been suggested [25].

Intracerebral Hematomas

Traumatic intracerebral hematomas may be defined as an intracerebrally confluent accumulation of blood. Differentiation from hemorrhagic contusions is arbitrary and reflects the amount of blood which can assume space-occupying dimensions. Often they seem to accumulate with time from contused brain tissue. This course of intracerebral hematomas, however, is at present unpredictable.

Some hematomas are not noted on the initial CT, while repeat CT hours or days later may demonstrate even large hematomas requiring surgical evacuation. Early traumaticintracerebral hematomas must be clearly distinguished from late diagnosis or delayed onset. The speculative phenomenon of *Spätapoplexie* described by Bollinger in 1891 [4] has not been verified by modern diagnostic methods. A small number of cases have been reported with an initially normal CT and genesis of a truly delayed intracerebral hematoma on the follow-up repeat CT after hours or days [9, 11, 13, 23, 30, 31].

The location of the intracerebral hematoma and preoperative neurological findings are undoubtedly of prognostic relevance. Mortality from traumatic hematomas of the posterior fossa ranges from 0% in clouding of consciousness to 82% in coma [14, 15].

Diagnosis

Any acute intracranial hematoma is best identified by CT. Contrast of an acute hematoma is undisputably less visible on MRI. Two days after the injury breakdown metabolites of the hematoma are detected by MRI, and even minute amounts of blood measuring less than 1 mm may be thus disclosed. Chronic subdural hematomas may be isodense on CT and can be identified after contrast enhancement or on MRI. In the absence of CT and MRI one may have to resort to exploratory burrholes or angiography. Timing is of paramount importance. Coma has been defined as the state of consciousness in which the patient cannot open his eyes and cannot obey commands [7, 18]. This may be equated with a Glasgow Coma Scale Score of 8 [33] or less.

Coma after head injury is by itself an urgent indicator for CT of the head. As epidural hematomas take some time to grow to a size causing a mass effect, and subdural hematomas in the first hour that have reached a size that cause a mass effect have practically no chance of survival, there is some initial time that may reasonably be spent for resuscitation, ventilation, and transportation. Ideally, however, it should not take more than 1 h until a cranial CT is obtained.

There may be a conflict of priorities in multiple injuries. Identification of an intracranial posttraumatic mass lesion may be delayed only in severe pulmonary or cardiovascular dysfunction.

Operative Measures

The type of surgery appears generall less important than its timing. Osteoplastic craniotomy is performed in epidural hematomas, and the bone removed often falls apart because of concomitant skull fracture. Stay sutures of the dura serve to pull the dura back into place and prevent recurrences.

With extreme brain swelling it may be warranted not to reinsert the bone flap. Acute subdural hematomas require a bone flap of suitable size as a clot rather than a liquid hematoma needs to be removed. In chronic subdural hematomas a twist drill or other types of hole and an external drainage is usually sufficient for rapid recovery.

Evacuation of intracerebral hematomas depends on the location and extent and is based on individual neurosurgical judgement. A microsurgical approach appears to be standard.

Endoscopic procedures are currently being tested for its efficacy. In 10 out of 289 initial CT scans after head injury (3.5 %) a confluent intracerebral hematoma was discovered 1–5 days after the injury [22]. Of these, 10 were operated upon. Only 4 of 120 contusions of immediate or delayed onset were forming confluent intracerebral hematomas that were judged to require surgical evacuation. Thus fewer than 5 % of patients with a head injury may be expected to require surgery for an intracerebral hematoma causing a mass effect.

Summary

Fractures. Diagnosis of fractures is based on plain skull X-ray or CT. Fractures of the skull usually require neurosurgical repair when they affect the vault, and depression causes a mass effect. Open head injuries need surgical repair to prevent late meningitis. Fractures of the midface should be operated upon when the patient is fit.

Intracranial Hematomas. The diagnostic tool of choice to identify an intracranial hematoma is CT. Coma, as the state of consciousness in which the patient cannot open the eyes and cannot obey commands, is an urgent indication for CT. No more than 1 h should be spent for intubation, resuscitation, and tranportation before performing CT of the comatose patient in a center where urgent neurosurgical care is available. Mortality of epidural hematomas increases with time after the injury and with the size of the hematoma. Mortality of subdural hematomas is related with the dynamics of the hematomas. Intracerebral hematomas causing a mass effect requiring surgery occur in approximately 3.5 % after head injury.

Clinical Guidelines. Coma is a state of consciousness in which the patient cannot open the eyes and cannot obey commands. The patient in coma after head injury must be intubated. No more than 1 h should be spent on intubation, resuscitation, and transportation before performing CT of the head to identify or exclude an intracranial hematoma in need of surgery.

References

1. Becker DP (1982) Acute subdural hematomas In: Vigouroux R (ed) Extracerebral collections. Advances in neurotraumatology, vol 1. Springer, Vienna New York, pp 51–100
2. Becker DP, Miller D, Greenberg R (1982) Prognosis after head injury. In: Youmans JR (ed) Neurological surgery, vol IV. Saunders, Philadelphia, pp 2137–2174
3. Bock WJ (1984) Schädel-Hirn-Verletzungen. In: Dietz H, Umbach W, Wüllenweber R (eds) Klinische Neurochirurgie, vol II. Thieme, Stuttgart
4. Bollinger O (1891) Über traumatische Spätapoplexie. Ein Beitrag zur Lehre von der Hirnerschütterung. In: Internationale Beiträge zur wissenschaftlichen Medizin. Festschrift Rudolf Virchow, vol 2. Hirschwald, Berlin, pp 459–470
5. Braakmann R, Jenett B (1976) Depressed skull fracture. In: Vinken P, Bruyn G (eds) Handbook of clinical neurology, vol 23. North Holland, Amsterdam, pp 403–414
6. Brihaye J (1986) Chronic subdural hematoma. In: Vigouroux R (ed) Advances in Neurotraumatology, extracerebral collections, vol 1. Springer, Vienna New York, pp 101–159
7. Brihaye J, Frowein RA, Lindgren S, Loew F, Stroobrandt G (1976) Report on the meeting of the WFNS Neurotraumatology Committee, Brussels, 19th–23rd of Sept. I. Coma scaling. Acta Neurochir (Wien) 40: 181–186
8. Brown F, Mullan S, Duda E (1978) Delayed traumatic intracerebral hematomas. J. Neurosurg 48: 1019–1022
9. Clifton G, Grossman R, Makela M, Miner M, Handel S, Sadhy V (1980) Neurological course and correlated computerized tomography findings after servere closed head injury. J Neurosurg 52: 611–624
10. Cooper PR (1987) Posttraumatic intracranial mass lesions. In: Cooper PR (ed) Head injury, 2nd edn. Williams and Wilkins, Baltimore
11. Diaz F, Kock D, Larson D, Rockswold G (1979) Early diagnosis of delayed posttraumatic intracerebral hematomas. J Neurosurg 50: 217–223
12. Dorfman L, Gaynon M, Ceranski J, Louis A, Howard J (1987) Visual electrical evoked potentials: evaluation of ocular injuries. Neurology 37: 123–128
13. Fernandez R, Firsching R, Lobato R, Mathiesen T, Pickard J, Servadei F, Tomei G, Brock M, Cohadon F, Rosenørn J (1997) Guidelines for treatment of head injury in adults. Opinions from a group of neurosurgeons. Zentralbl Neurochir (in press)
14. Firsching R, Frowein RA, Thun F (1987) Intracerebellar hematoma: eleven traumatic cases and a review of the literature. Neurochirurgia 30: 182–185
15. Firsching R, Steinbrich W, Thun F, Frowein RA (1987) CT-Zisternogramm zur Diagnose nasaler Liquorfisteln. Akt Traumatol 17: 187–192
16. Firsching R, Frowein RA, Thun F (1989) Encapsulated subdural hematoma. Neurosurg Rev 12 [Suppl 1]: 207–214
17. Firsching R, Heimann M, Frowein RA (1997) Early dynamics of acute extradural and subdural hematomas. Neurol Res (in press)
18. Frowein RA (1976) Classification of coma. Acta Neurochir (Wien)34: 5–10
19. Frowein RA, Firsching R (1990) Classification of head injury In: Braakman R (ed) Handbook of clinical Neurology, vol 13. Elsevier, Amsterdam, pp 101–122
20. Frowein RA, Karimi-Nejad A, Nittner K, Pachay R, Richard K-E, Steinmann W, Terhaag R (1977) Verletzungen des Kopfes In: Zenker R, Deucher F, Schink W (eds) Chirurgie der Gegenwart, vol 4a. Urban und Schwarzberg, Munich, pp 2–80
21. Frowein RA, Keila M (1972) Einteilung der traumatischen subduralen Hämatome. Akt Traumatol 4: 205–213

22. Frowein RA, Stammler U, Firsching R, Friedmann G, Thun F (1991) Early dynamic evolution of cerebral contusions and lacerations. Clinical and radiological findings. In: Frowein RA (ed) Advances in neurotraumatology. Cerebral contusions, lacerations and hematoms, vol 3. Springer, Vienna New York, pp 201–228
23. Fukamachi A, Nagaseki Y, Kohno K, Wakao T (1985) The incidence and developmental progress of delayed traumatic intracerebral hematomas. Acta Neurochir (Wien) 74: 35–39
24. Jamieson KG, Yelland J (1968) Extradural hematoma, report of 167 cases J Neurosurg 29: 13–23
25. Jennett B, Teasdale G (1981) Management of head injuries. Davis, Philadelphia
26. Lobato R, Rivas J, Cordobes F, Alted E, Perez C, Sarabia R, Cabera A, Diez I, Gomez P, Lamas E (1988) Acute epidural hematoma: an analysis of factors influencing the outcome of patients undergoing surgery in coma. J Neurosurgery 68: 48–57
27. Loew F, Pertuiset B, Chaumier F., Jacksche H (1984) Traumatic, spontaneous and postoperative CSF. Rhinorrhea, In: Symon L et al (eds) Advances and technical standards. Neurosurgery, vol 11. Springer Berlin Heidelberg New York, pp 169–207
28. Meirowsky AM (1965) Compound fractures of the convexity of the skull. Neurological surgery of trauma. Government Printing Office, Washington, pp 83–101
29. Mendelow AD, Teasdale G, Jennett B, Bryden J, Hessett C, Murray G (1983) Risks of intracranial hematoma in head injured adults. BMJ 287: 1173–1176 .
30. Nanassis K, Frowein RA, Karini A, Thun F (1989) Delayed posttraumatic intracerebral bleeding Neurosurg Rev 12 [Suppl 1]: 243–251
31. Ninchoji T, Kemura K, Shinoyama J, Hinokuma K, Bun T, Nakjima S (1984) Traumatic intracerebral hematomas of delayed onset. In: Acta Neurochir (Wien) 71: 69–90
32. Richards T, Hoff J (1974) Factors affecting survival from acute subdural hematoma. Surgery 75: 253–258
33. Teasdale G, Jennett B (1974) Assesment of coma and impaired cousciousness. Lancet 2: 81–84
34. Thomas L, Gurdjian E (1973) Intracranial hematomas of traumatic origin. In: Youmans J (ed) Neurological surgery, vol II. Philadelphia, Saunders, pp 960–968
35. Voris H (1941) The diagnosis and treatment of subdural hematomas. Surgery 10: 447–456
36. Williams J, Gomes G, Drudge O, Kessler M (1984) Predicting outcome from closed head injury by early assessment of trauma severity. J Neurosurg 61: 581–585

9 Panfacial Fractures

W. Hochban

Introduction

The chances of survival for patients with severe brain injuries have improved considerably in recent years. Brain injuries are often combined with fractures of the facial skeleton which – in contrast to the brain injuries – are life-threatening only in rare cases. Bleeding from the cranial base can be stopped by tamponage, for example, and airway obstruction in cases with mandibular fractures is nonthreatening due to endotracheal intubation. Unfortunately, the correct diagnosis of fractures of the viscerocranium is sometimes delayed, and immediate proper treatment is hindered. Occasionally, minor injuries such as isolated zygomatic fractures or closed fractures of the temporomandibular joint are not recognized at all. For the patient who survives, the sequelae of these fractures are of major importance, not only with respect to esthetics but also to functional disturbances. Due to the complex structure of the viscerocranium, minor dislocations may cause major disturbances. Whereas secondary soft tissue corrections may yield good results, skeletal deformities are much more difficult to be corrected secondarily and often cause severe defacement.

Unfortunately, continuous specialization has led to less knowledge about the peculiarities of craniomaxillofacial injuries among the other disciplines.

Methods

The definition of panfacial fractures is not commonly accepted. Dividing the viscerocranium into six traumatological areas (frontal, frontobasal, orbital, nasal, maxillary, mandibulary), a fracture is sometimes defined as panfacial if only two out of the six are involved [5]. To be classified as "panfacial" an injury must normally involve the upper, middle, and lower face with the naso-orbital ethmoidal structures, the the zygomatic complex, the Le Fort midfacial area, and the mandible [3, 6].

Over the 2-year period of 1994–1996, 73 polytraumatized patients with complex midfacial fractures were treated at the craniomaxillofacial unit of the Philipps University in Marburg. Only 16 of these 73 patients had complete panfacial fractures with involvement of all the frontobasal, periorbital, nasomaxillary areas and the mandible. More than 90 % of our 73 patients had accompanying severe brain injuries.

Despite the mandatory wearing of seat belts and the introduction of the air bag vehicular accidents are the most common etiological factors in our clientele. However, in comparison to previous years there has been an increasing number of severe facial injuries due to sports-related accidents, especially bicycling.

Normally the unconscious injured patient is admitted to the hospital with an oral endotracheal intubation. For the reconstruction of the midfacial pillars it is essential to reestablish and maintain the dental occlusion [2, 3, 5]. This means the maxillary and mandibulary arches must be realigned. The recreated preinjury dental occlusal relationship must be maintained by arch bars and – at least during the surgical bony reconstruction – by maxillomandibulary fixation. Therefore a nasal endotracheal intubation is mandatory. A tracheostomy is not used as first-line therapy in cases with pan-/midfacial fractures. The decision for a tracheostomy should be postponed until the complete extent of the injury is visible among the various disciplines, and performed only if brain or lung injuries demand a long-term intubation and respiration.

A few cases with major soft tissue injuries demand immediate reconstruction of the underlying skeletal fractures, often without sufficient radiological examination prior to surgery. In these cases osteosynthesis must be applied only in respect to clinical symptoms and knowledge of expected designated sites of facial fractures (as described by Le Fort at the turn of the century; Fig. 1).

Other cases with severe brain injuries and accompaning edema may not permit immediate surgery. If ever possible, reconstruction in panfacial fractures should be accomplished within the first 5 – 10 days. If the surgical reconstruction of the face must be postponed longer than 14 days, functional disturbances are often the consequences, especially in respect to eye motility.

Cranial computed tomography (CCT) is mandatory due to the brain injury. A CT of the viscerocranium should be obtained at the same time, which is the

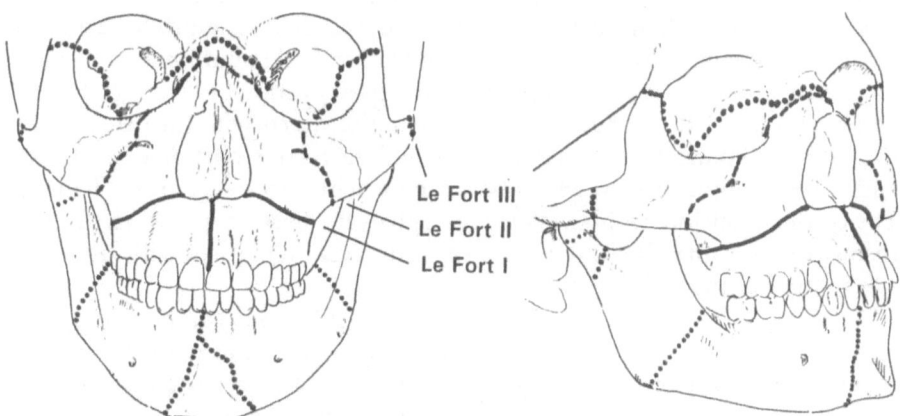

Fig. 1. Common sites of midfacial and mandibular fractures

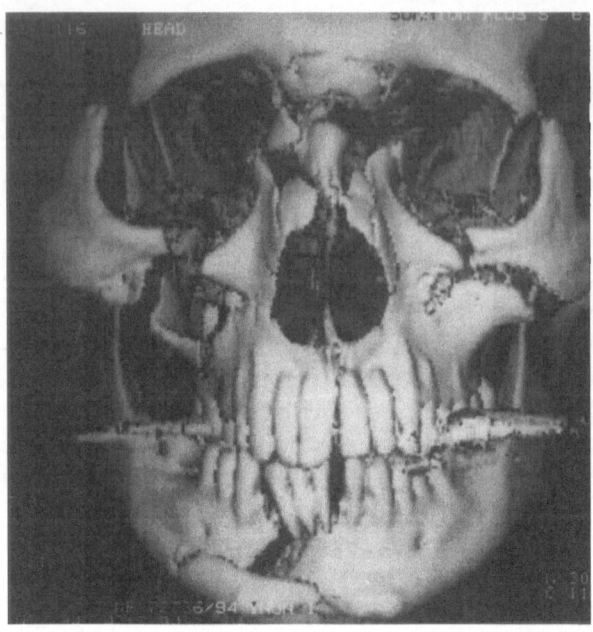

Fig. 2. Panfacial fracture with injury to the frontobasal, periorbital, nasomaxillary, and mandibular region. The midfacial injuries may be classified as bilateral Le Fort I, II, and III fractures with sagittal fracture of the maxilla. The mandible is transversely widened

most useful modality and reveals the best information about complex facial injuries. A three-dimensional CT may help to better understand the comminution in panfacial fractures (Fig. 2).

Reestablishing the facial appearance and function in its complex three dimensions of width, height and projection means reconstruction of the bony pillars or buttresses vertically and horizontally. Two principle surgical strategies are used: The first method begins with the reconstruction of the mandible with rigid internal fixation. The reestablished dental arch (at least in dentulous patients) is the base for further reconstruction of the vertical nasofrontal, zygomaticomaxillary, and pterygopalatal midfacial buttresses. These vertical pillars are connected by horizontal struts at the skull base, supra- and infraorbital rim, zygomatic arch, palatal plate, and horizontal mandibular arch which must also be reconstructed properly for the preservation of facial width.

The second method of surgical reconstruction starts with the osteosynthesis of the zygomatic processes to the skull and the reconstruction of the frontal and nasoethmoidal bones, which best can be achieved via a coronal incision. The coronal incision avoids visible scars, gives the best overview for the bony reconstruction, and allows the neurosurgical revision in cases with large injuries to the frontobasal region.

Fixation of fractures at the frontozygomatic processes can best be accomplished with miniplates, whereas thinner bony structures as in the nasofrontal region and the zygomatic arches usually are fixed with microplates [2]. Both mini- and microplates are suited in the midfacial region according to the thickness of the bony fragments. Miniplates are also used for the rigid internal

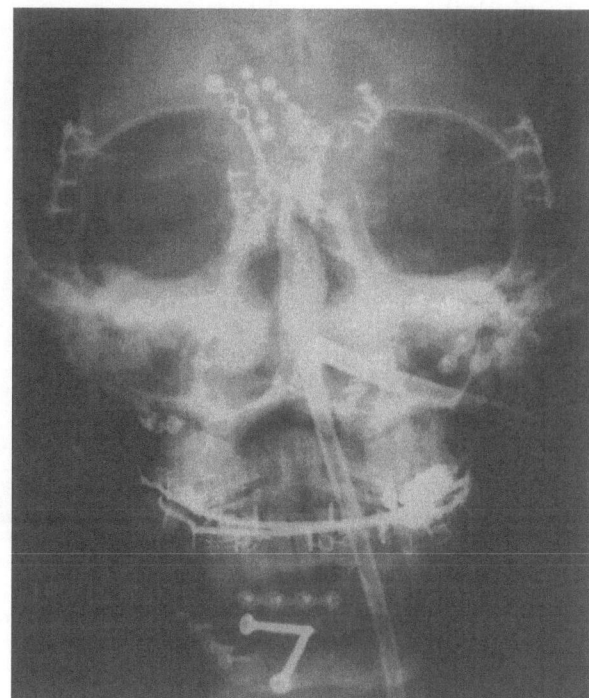

Fig. 3. Panfacial fracture (same patient as in Fig. 2) immediately after open reduction, frontobasal revision, and internal rigid fixation with mini- and microplates and oblique lag screw osteosynthesis in the fronto-mandibular region for compensation of transverse widening of the mandible

fixation of the mandible. Due to their weakness of bending strength across the plane surface, miniplates are not suited for bending fractures of the corpus mandibulae. These fractures of the mandible are characterized by transverse widening of the mandible and are best kept by lag screw fixation to avoid transverse widening of the lower face (Fig. 3).

Results

Most of our patients were treated on this basis within 1 week after the injury if the severe brain injury did allow surgical intervention at that stage. During the 2-year period 73 patients with complex midfacial injuries were treated. According to our definition, only 16 of the 73 patients had a complete panfacial fracture with the frontobasal, periorbital, nasomaxillary, and mandibular bones involved. In 19 patients with frontobasal fractures, lacerations of the dura were closed simultaneously. Secondary rhinoliquorrhea did not occur in any case due to the immediate reconstruction with internal rigid fixation.

Secondary bony corrections were not necessary except in two cases: one of the patients needed a maxillary Le Fort I osteotomy for correction of malocclusion, and a second patient lost one-third of the maxilla by the accident,

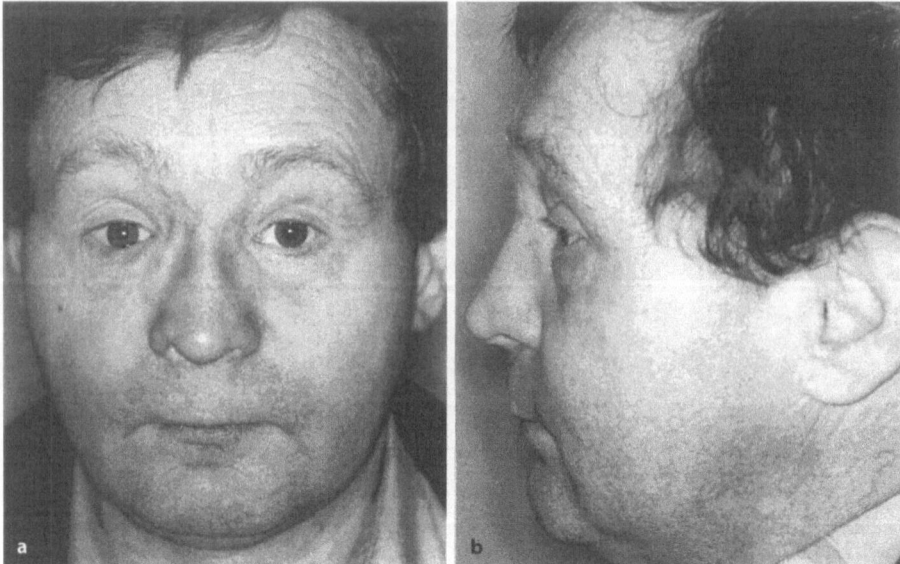

Fig. 4a,b. Panfacial fracture (same patient as in Figs. 2, 3) a few months after treatment without any further secondary corrections. **a** Frontal view. **b** Profile

which had to be reconstructed by a secondary bone grafting. Figure 4 shows an example of a patient (the same patient as Fig. 2) 6 months after treatment of a panfacial fracture without any secondary corrections at that time. Diplopia did not occur in any case, but three patients had lost nearly complete vision in one eye by the injury, and therefore binocular vision could not be controlled in these three patients postoperatively. There was a complete restoration of eye motility in all other patients.

Discussion

There is of course no question that life-threatening injuries such as severe brain injuries have priority over the treatment of facial fractures [4]. Nevertheless, for the patients who survive the facial appearance and configuration is important not only for many organs (especially for the proper function of the eyes) but also for their personal identity. Soft tissue injuries may cause scaring but usually do not lead to the loss of identity. Scars can often be corrected secondarily with good results. The displacement and dislocation even of smaller parts of the bony skeleton may completely change facial appearance and thus alter the identity of a person. Fragments of the facial skeleton can soon consolidate even in a malposition, secondary bony corrections are much more difficult to perform and often present unsatisfying results. Therefore early reduction and fixation of the bony fragments within a period of 5–10 days should be always aspired for. This also holds true for patients with severe brain injuries even if the chance of survival cannot always be judged in advance with certainty.

Open reduction and internal rigid fixation is the method of choice for the treatment of panfacial and midfacial as well as mandibular fractures. Fronto-maxillary wire suspension should no longer be used due to the incorrect positioning of the midface with dorsocranial displacement. Mini- and microplates even allow the restoration of minor defects and bony dislocations, which is especially helpful in the reconstruction of the thin bones around the paranasal sinuses. Fewer infections occur. Also, the incidence of rhinoliquorrhea with secondary infections is reduced, due to the rigid internal fixation. Although this surgical procedure is time consuming (especially in complete panfacial fractures with involvement of all parts of the face), it is worthwhile for the functional reasons and for the preservation of the facial appearance and configuration.

Summary

Patients with severe panfacial fractures usually also have severe brain injuries. Despite the uncertainty of survival of patients with severe brain injury, surgical reconstruction of the facial fractures should be performed within 5–10 days to yield good results. Open reduction and internal rigid fixation is the method of choice for the treatment of panfacial fractures. Mini- and microplates allow the precise three-dimensional reconstruction of the facial skeleton. There is sometimes the need for the additional use of more stable reconstruction plates or lag screw osteosynthesis in the mandible. Rigid internal fixation is not only important for the proper function of the various organs in the viscerocranium, but also for the facial appearance and the identity of the person after recovery from the accident.

References

1. Kelly KJ, Manson PN, van der Kolk CA, Markowitz BL, Dunham CM, Rumley TO, Crawley WA (1990) Sequencing Le Fort fracture treatment: organization of treatment for a panfacial fracture. J Craniofac Surg 1: 168–178
2. Luhr HG (1991) Plattenosteosynthese in der Traumatologie des Mittelgesichts: ein Fortschritt? Fortschr Kiefergesichtschir 36: 3630–3633
3. Markowitz BL, Manson PN (1989) Panfacial fractures: organization of treatment. Clin Plast Surg 16: 105–114
4. Metelmann HR, Waite P, Kindermann H, Hannemann L, Rudolph KH (1991) Operationszeitpunkt und Hirndrucksenkung bei Patienten mit schweren kraniomaxillofazialen Unfallverletzungen. Fortschr Kiefergesichtschir 36: 42–43
5. Schilli W, Joos U (1991) Behandlung panfazialer Frakturen. Fortschr Kiefergesichtschir 36: 36–38
6. Wenig BL (1991) Management of panfacial fractures. Otolaryngol Clin North Am 24: 93–101

10 Cerebral Blood Flow, Hyperventilation, and Metabolism in Severe Head Injury

D.W. Marion

Introduction

The functional outcome of a patient who suffers severe traumatic brain injury (TBI) is in large part determined by the degree of physiological and metabolic damage that occurs in the first few hours and days following the injury. As basic science investigations reveal the complex physiological and metabolic abnormalities that result from trauma to the brain, methods of treating these abnormalities are being developed and have already have been shown to improve outcome. While many of the mechanisms responsible for secondary brain injury have yet to be identified, it is increasingly apparent that ischemia plays a fundamental role.

Cerebral Blood Flow Changes Resulting From Traumatic Brain Injury

Following trauma to the brain that is severe enough to cause loss of consciousness there is a sharp decline in cerebral blood flow (CBF). In prospective studies of these patients the CBF during the first 8 h after injury is usually less than 30 ml 100 g^{-1} min^{-1}, and may be less than 25 ml 100 g^{-1} min^{-1} during the first 4 h of injury [5, 6, 20]. There is evidence that a sustained CBF of 17 ml 100 g^{-1} min^{-1} or less leads to irreversible ischemia and infarction [15].

In addition to the global CBF reduction, there is significant regional heterogeneity in this reduction of flow following severe TBI. Thus CBF within a contusion is significantly less than that surrounding the contusion, and both of these CBF values are often significantly lower than mean global CBF [7]. The CBF in the brain tissue underlying an acute subdural hematoma is also significantly lower than global CBF and may remain low even after the subdural hematoma has been evacuated [33].

Traumatic brain injury also causes changes in the normal physiological response of the cerebral vasculature to alterations in blood pressure (pressure autoregulation) and the arterial CO_2 tension (CO_2 vasoresponsivity) [4, 8, 34]. Early after severe TBI many patients have a passive increase or decrease in CBF, with corresponding changes in the systemic blood pressure [4]. Normal individuals regulate CBF within a very narrow range throughout a wide range of blood pressures, and it therefore appears that trauma causes loss of pressure autoregulation in these cases. In addition, the cerebral vasculature normally constricts in response to a reduction of arterial CO_2 tension at a rate sufficient to cause a 3% decrease in CBF per torr change in the pCO_2. Following trauma the global average value of this effect is often unchanged, but there is significant regional heterogeneity [19]. The CO_2 vasoresponsivity within or surrounding contusions may vary from 0% to 9% [23]. Such changes are difficult to predict for individual patients but do appear to be more common and more severe in those with the most severe injuries.

The significance of these abnormalities is not completely understood. While the typical CBF early after injury appears to be dangerously close to the threshold for irreversible ischemia (17 ml 100 g^{-1} min^{-1}), this may not always be a critical threshold for comatose victims of TBI. Obrist et al. [27] have reported that the cerebral metabolic rate for oxygen in patients with severe TBI is typically less than 50% of the rate for normal people. Since the level of CBF that causes ischemia depends on the metabolic demands of the tissue, their findings suggest that the traumatized brain should tolerate CBF levels much lower than normal. They suggest that the low CBF levels seen following TBI may be appropriate for the level of posttraumatic cerebral metabolism, and that a higher CBF would actually indicate uncoupling of CBF with metabolism and represent hyperemia. Good recoveries have been documented in patients with global or regional CBF values as low as 10 ml 100 g^{-1} min^{-1} [9]. Such cases are particularly common when the CBF is reduced during therapeutic moderate hypothermia or barbiturate therapy [21]. The significance of loss of pressure autoregulation and CO_2 vasoresponsivity also is not clear. While there does appear to be an association with the loss of these variables and the severity of brain injury, good outcomes can occur following their loss [8].

Metabolic Changes Resulting From Traumatic Brain Injury

Cerebral ischemia induces a number of metabolic events that can result in damage to capillary endothelium and cell membranes, and ultimately lead to cell death [29]. Ischemia results in the depletion of high-energy molecular stores used by many of the cell membrane-associated enzyme systems responsible for maintaining the physiological balance of intra- and extracellular electrolytes such as calcium, sodium, and potassium [24]. Disruption of this balance leads to cell swelling and death. Ischemia may also be responsible for the accumulation of high levels of extracellular excitatory amino acids such as glutamate. Glutamate is a potent agonist of the N-methyl D-aspartate family of receptors which can enhance calcium transport into the cell [32]. High levels of intracellular calcium mediate several biochemical reactions leading to the production of oxygen free radicals. An excess of free radicals lyses cell membranes, disrupts the blood brain barrier, and even promotes the release of more glutamate [14]. High levels of glutamate have been measured in the extracellular space using in vivo microdialysis, and in the ventricular CSF following severe TBI. Recently it was found that ventricular CSF levels of glutamate increase for at least the first 3 – 4 days after injury, suggesting that there is ongoing secondary brain injury for the first several days after trauma [28].

Several other mechanisms of formation of free radicals also have been identified. Iron released from intracellular stores or from the breakdown of hemoglobin participates in several reactions responsible for the production of superoxide and hydroxyl radicals [16]. Iron also is a potent promoter of lipid peroxidation. Superoxide and nitric oxide are produced by several cellular components of the central nervous system following ischemia, and these two species can combine to form the peroxynitrite anion, a molecule that is metabolized to form the hydroxyl radical [2].

TBI also leads to the release of cytokines, one of the more important of which is interleukin-1b [26]. Interleukin-1b is involved in central temperature regulation, but it also is important in initiating the inflammatory response following trauma. This cytokine has potent leukostatic properties and can enhance the migration of leukocytes across the blood-brain barrier. High levels of interleukin-lb appear in the ventricular CSF within hours after injury and remain for several days [22]. Other members of the interleukin family also appear to play a role in secondary brain injury, although their role is not yet understood [37].

Many of the clinical investigations attempting to define the incidence of posttraumatic ischemia have focused on oxygen utilization by the damaged brain. In some centers the use of oxygen by the brain is routinely monitored by placing a catheter or probe into the jugular bulb and determining the oxygen saturation or oxygen content of the blood after it passes through the brain [35]. These studies indicate that there is an increase in oxygen extraction early after injury, at a time when CBF is the lowest [5]. There also appears to be a correlation between the increase in oxygen extraction and the severity of brain injury, as well as the neurological outcome [30]. Recently it has been suggested that glucose metabolism is even more critical than oxygen metabolism in determining the detrimental effects of ischemia. Several experimental studies of TBI reveal a significant increase in glucose utilization by the damaged brain early after injury [1, 17], and there is some evidence that ischemic brain injury can be lessened if glucose is provided, even in the face of hypoxemia [36]. The increase in glucose utilization following trauma may be related to a posttraumatic increase in extracellular potassium.

Implications for Treatment: Hyperventilation

Reduction of the arterial tension of carbon dioxide with the use of artificial hyperventilation, usually facilitated by endotracheal intubation, has long been a cornerstone in the management of patients with severe TBI. More than 40 years ago, and shortly after the development of intracranial pressure (ICP) monitoring techniques, it was observed that hyperventilation is a rapid and effective method of reducing elevated ICP in many patients with intracranial hypertension [18]. This therapy has since become one of the most commonly used to manage elevated ICP. Some have even advocated the prophylactic use of hyperventilation therapy and maintain an arterial pCO_2 of 25 – 28 mm Hg for the first several days after injury in the belief that this prevents brain swelling.

However, there is increasing evidence to suggest that hypocapneic therapy is not appropriate for most patients with severe TBI, particularly during the first 24 – 36 h after injury. Because CBF typically is low during the first few hours after severe TBI, and if it is effective, hypocapneic therapy must lower the CBF even further, there is a risk of inducing ischemia with this therapy. In a rodent model of controlled cortical contusion we compared the extent of brain tissue injury and functional deficits in animals kept at an arterial pCO_2 of 20 mm Hg for 5 h after injury vs. animals kept at an arterial pCO_2 of 35 mm Hg (normocapneic) during that same time [12]. When killed 14 days after injury, the normocapneic animals had a significantly higher number of surviving neurons in the CA3 region of the hippocampus than did the hyperventilated animals. However, there was no difference between the groups in Morris Water maze performance or in the size of the contusion.

Gopinath et al. [13] measured the incidence of jugular venous oxygen desaturations (O_2 saturation < 50%) in a series of patients with severe TBI and found that poor neurological outcomes were directly correlated with the incidence and duration of desaturations. Importantly, however, they found that hypocapnia was the second most common identifiable cause for jugular venous desaturations [35].

Because of the regional heterogeneity of CO_2 vasoresponsivity, the risk of causing regional ischemia with hyperventilation therapy seems even greater. For example, a patient with a hemorrhagic contusion is likely to have an area of the contusion which contains dead tissue, and within thist tissue the vessels lose all ability to regulate their diameter and are maximally dilated. In a 2- to 3-cm rim of tissue surrounding the contusion the brain may be ischemic, and often the vessels in ischemic tissue have abnormally high CO_2 vasoresponsivity [7]. Treating such a patient with hypocapneic therapy is likely to severely increase the resistance of the vessels in the ischemic zone of brain surrounding the contusion and shunt blood into the low resistance vessels within the dead portion of the contusion. The end result of this is exacerbation of ischemia in the brain tissue that may have otherwise recovered, and exacerbation of brain swelling by shunting unnecessary blood into maximally dilated vessels.

The use of hyperventilation therapy to reduce ICP is based on the assumption that this therapy leads to a decrease in cerebral blood volume, since it is the cerebral blood volume and not the CBF that is directly related to ICP. However, hyperventilation therapy has a direct effect only on CBF. Bouma and Muizellar [3] measured CBF and cerebral blood volume simultaneously in a series of patients with severe TBI and found that no significant correlation between the two. Their findings confirmed the clinical observations of most neurosurgeons that patients with severe TBI respond to hyperventilation therapy in a very unpredictable way. The reduction in CBF caused by this therapy is far more predictable, however.

Hyperventilation therapy has not been convincingly shown to cause ischemia or infarction in patients with severe TBI, but clinical evidence suggests that its prophylactic use can lead to worse neurological outcomes. A prospective randomized trial assigned patients with severe TBI either to a group with an arterial pCO_2 kept at 25 mm Hg for 5 days following injury or to a group kept at 35 mm Hg during for the same period [25]. Those with lower pCO_2 had a significantly worse outcome at 3 and 6 months after injury than those with higher pCO_2. Outcomes were similar 1 year after injury, but attrition in the number of patients available for follow-up may have been responsible for this. Several clinical studies have subsequently found significantly better outcomes than in historical controls with the use of acute care protocols that emphasize the maintenance of normal or near normal pCO_2 levels [21, 31].

Some have advocated the use of hyperventilation therapy to "normalize" cerebral oxygen or glucose metabolism following severe TBI [10, 11]. By determining the difference between the simultaneously obtained jugular venous and arterial contents of these metabolites they suggest that this difference is brought closer to published norms for these values with the use of hyperventilation therapy. This reasoning is flawed in two important ways. First, the published norms for the arterial jugular venous differences in oxygen or glucose contents refer to normal individuals, and there is abundant clinical evidence demonstrating significant global and regional alterations of metabolism following severe TBI. Secondly, at best the content of metabolites in jugular venous blood represents a mix of the metabolites produced in areas of the brain that are hypo- or hypermetabolic. Jugular venous sampling is insensitive to regional metabolic abnormalities.

Contemporary management of patients with severe TBI must account for the regional heterogeneity of posttraumatic metabolic and physiological derangements if we are to improve functional outcomes in these patients. Based on the regional abnormalities of CBF and CO_2 vasoresponsivity that we and others have demonstrated it seems short-sighted to use a therapy such has aggressive hyperventilation in most patients with severe TBI since there is the potential for worsening regional ischemia in eloquent areas of the brain. Therapies such as mannitol, cerebrospinal fluid drainage, barbiturates, and hypothermia often can provide the desired reduction in ICP through mechanisms that may actually benefit the injured brain and may therefore be preferable to hyperventilation.

References

1. Andersen BJ, Marmarou A (1992) Post-traumatic selective stimulation of glycolysis. Brain Res 585: 184–189
2. Beckman JS, Beckman TW, Chen J et al (1990) Apparent hydroxyl radical production by peroxynitrite: implications for endothelial injury from nitric oxide and superoxide. Proc Natl Acad Sci USA 87: 1620–1624
3. Bouma GJ, Muizelaar JP (1992) Cerebral blood flow, cerebral blood volume, and cerebrovascular reactivity after severe head injury. J Neurotrauma 9: S333–S348
4. Bouma GJ, Muizelaar JP, Bandoh K et al (1992) Blood pressure and intracranial pressure-volume dynamics in severe head injury: relationship with cerebral blood flow. J Neurosurg 77: 15–19
5. Bouma GJ, Muizelaar JP, Choi SC et al (1991) Cerebral circulation and metabolism after severe traumatic brain injury: the elusive role of ischemia. J Neurosurg 75: 685–693
6. Bouma GJ, Muizelaar JP, Stringer WA et al (1992) Ultra-early evaluation of regional cerebral blood flow in severely head-injured patients using xenon-enhanced computerized tomography. J Neurosurg 77: 360–368
7. Bullock R, Sakas D, Patterson J et al (1992) Early post-traumatic cerebral blood flow mapping: correlation with structural damage after focal injury. Acta Neurochir Suppl (Wien) 55: 14–17
8. Cold GE (1989) Measurements of CO_2 reactivity and barbiturate reactivity in patients with severe head injury. Acta Neurochir (Wien) 98: 153–163
9. Cruz J (1994) Low clinical ischemic threshold for cerebral blood flow in severe acute brain trauma. Case report. J Neurosurg 80: 143–147
10. Cruz J (1995) An additional therapeutic effect of adequate hyperventilation in severe acute brain trauma: normalization of cerebral glucose uptake. J Neurosurg 82: 379–385
11. Cruz J, Gennarelli TA, Hoffstad OJ (1992) Lack of relevance of the Bohr effect in optimally ventilated patients with acute brain trauma (discusion). J Trauma 33: 304–10
12. Forbes ML, Clark RSB, Dixon CE et al (1997) Hyperventilation early after traumatic brain injury in rats augments neuronal death in CA3 hippocampus. J Crit Care Med (Abstr) 25: 2–19
13. Gopinath SP, Robertson CS, Contant CF et al (1994) Jugular venous desaturation and outcome after head injury. J Neurol Neurosurg Psychiatry 57: 717–723
14. Hall ED (1993) The role of oxygen radicals in traumatic injury: clinical implications. J Emerg Med 11: 31–36
15. Heiss WD, Huber M, Fink GR et al (1992) Progressive derangement of periinfarct viable tissue in ischemic stroke. J Cereb Blood Flow Metab 12: 193–203
16. Kontos HA (1989) Oxygen radicals in CNS damage. Chem Biol Int 72: 229–255
17. Kuroda Y, Inglis FM, Miller JD et al (1992) Transient glucose hypermetabolism after acute subdural hematoma in the rat. J Neurosurg 76: 471–477
18. Lundberg N, Kjallquist A, Bien C (1959) Reduction of increased intracranial pressure by hyperventilation. Acta Psychiatr Scand 34: 4–64
19. Marion DW, Bouma GJ (1991) The use of stable xenon-enhanced computed tomographic studies of cerebral blood flow to define changes in cerebral carbon dioxide vasoresponsivity caused by a severe head injury. Neurosurg 29: 869–873
20. Marion DW, Darby J, Yonas H (1991) Acute regional cerebral blood flow changes caused by severe head injuries. J Neurosurg 74: 407–414
21. Marion DW, Obrist WD, Carlier PM et al (1993) The use of moderate therapeutic hypothermia for patients with severe head injuries: a preliminary report. J Neurosurg 79: 354–362
22. McClain CJ, Cohen D, Ott L et al (1987) Ventricular fluid interleukin-1 activity in patients with head injury. J Lab Clin Med 110: 48–54
23. McLaughlin MR, Marion DW (1996) Cerebral blood flow and vasoresponsivity within and around cerebral contusions. J Neurosurg 85: 871–876
24. Miller JD (1985) Head injury and brain ischaemia – implications for therapy. Br J Anaesth 57: 120–130
25. Muizelaar JP, Marmarou A, Ward JD et al (1991) Adverse effects of prolonged hyperventilation in patients with severe head injury: A randomized clinical trial. J Neurosurg 75: 731–739

26. Negro A, Tavella A, Facci L et al (1992) Interleukin-1 beta regulates proenkephalin gene expression in astrocytes cultured from rat cortex. Glia 6: 206–212
27. Obrist WD, Langfitt TW, Jaggi JL et al (1984) Cerebral blood flow and metabolism in comatose patients with acute head injury. J Neurosurg 61: 241–253
28. Palmer AM, Marion DW, Botscheller ML et al (1994) Increased transmitter amino acid concentration in human ventricular CSF posttrauma. Neuroreport 6: 153–156
29. Robertson CS, Clifton GL, Grossman RG et al (1988) Alterations in cerebral availability of metabolic substrates after severe head injury. J Trauma 28: 1523–1532
30. Robertson CS, Contant CF, Gokaslan ZL et al (1992) Cerebral blood flow, arteriovenous oxygen difference, and outcome in head injured patients. J Neurol Neurosurg Psychiatry 55: 594–603
31. Rosner MJ, Rosner SD, Johnson AH (1995) Cerebral perfusion pressure: management protocol and clinical results. J Neurosurg 83: 949–962
32. Saito N, Chang C, Kawai K et al (1990) Role of neuroexcitation in development of blood-brain barrier and oedematous changes following cerebral ischaemia and traumatic brain injury. Acta Neurochir Suppl (Wien) 51: 186–188
33. Salvant JB, Muizelaar JP (1993) Changes in cerebral blood flow and metabolism related to the presence of subdural hematoma. Neurosurg 33: 387–393
34. Saunders ML, Miller JD, Stablein D et al (1979) The effects of graded experimental trauma on cerebral blood flow and responsiveness to CO2. J Neurosurg 51: 18–26
35. Sheinberg M, Kanter MJ, Robertson CS et al (1992) Continuous monitoring of jugular venous oxygen saturation in head-injured patients. J Neurosurg 76: 212–217
36. Swanson RA, Chen J, Graham SH (1994) Glucose can fuel glutamate uptake in ischemic brain. J Cereb Blood Flow Metab 14: 1–6
37. Yan HQ, Banos MA, Herregodts P et al (1992) Expression of interleukin (IL)-1 beta, IL-6 and their respective receptors in the normal rat brain and after injury. Eur J Immunol 22: 2963–2971

11 Management of Intracranial Hypertension in Pediatric Head Injury

M.J. Fritsch, K.H. Manwaring, and D.H. Beyda

Introduction

The mortality associated with severe head injury seems to be lower for children than for adults. Luerssen found a mortality of 28 % in children presenting with a Glascow Coma Score (GCS) of 3 – 8 compared to a mortality of 48 % in adults presenting with the same GCS range [25]. Lang compared mortality in adults and children with posttraumatic brain swelling. The mortality in adults was higher with 35 % than the 20 % found in children with brain swelling [40]. The three major causes of brain injury in children are falls, motor vehicle accidents and bicycle accidents [33].

Brain injury occurs in two phases. The primary injury is due to a mechanic damage that happens at the time of the insult and the secondary injury is the result of hypoxia, increased intracranial pressure and decreased cerebral blood flow. An understanding of these secondary pathophysiologic changes in time after the injury is important to provide head-injured children with intracranial hypertension with appropriate treatment.

Pathophysiologic Changes in Time After Severe Head Injury in Children

Cerebral Blood Flow

Normal global cerebral blood flow (CBF) values range around a mean value of 65 ml/100 g per minute in children [8] and 42 ml/100 g per minute in newborns [14]. Normal mean global CBF in awake young adults ranges around 44 ml/100 g per minute [7]. Hyperemia was defined as CBF above normal blood flow plus two standard deviations [17]. There is a wide variation in CBF in similar pediatric patients with head injury and also within the same patient over time [35]. It must be considered that CBF values vary depending on the type of injury and that global measurements do not reflect the local blood flow accurately [11, 39].

CBF within brain contusions seems to be reduced relative to surrounding parenchyma [45, 50].

Head injured children present with a low normal or reduced global CBF in the early hours postinjury and develop a hyperemic state by 38 – 72 h postinjury [27, 48]. There is no significant difference between adults and children in the response of cerebral blood flow after severe head injury. Studies in adults have shown that in patients without surgical mass lesion the CBF within the first hours after injury is low, followed by a hyperemic phase that is significant at 24–72 h postinjury [3, 31, 32].

Sharples found a initial presentation with a blood flow below the normal values in 77 % of her pediatric patients and a non significant increase in CBF in time postinjury [46]. In the first 24 h mean CBF is significantly higher in patients with good or moderate outcome than in patients with poor outcome [46].

In children initial CBF tends to be lower with low GCS scores and hyperemia tends to be more significant in the same group [27]. The severest injured patients with a GCS of 3 do not follow this pattern and have a low global CBF [27].

Arterial Venous Oxygen Difference (AVDO₂)

Normal $AVDO_2$ in children at a PCO_2 of 40 mm Hg is 6.3 vol % [1]. In children with severe head injury the $AVDO_2$ falls significantly between the first and the third day after injury [46]. A low $AVDO_2$ together with a normal or elevated CBF is also found in the majority of adult patients who developed intracranial hypertension [17]. If the CBF is functionally coupled with brain metabolism the occurrence of high blood flow and low oxygen demand suggests uncoupling of blood flow and metabolism [27, 48]. $AVDO_2$ tends to be closer to normal as GCS scores increases. Initial low $AVDO_2$ seems to be a bad prognostic sign.

Cerebral Metabolic Rate for Oxygen (CMRO₂)

The $CMRO_2$ is determined by the CBF and the $AVDO_2$ in the following way: $CMRO_2 = CBF$ times $AVDO_2$. Normal $CMRO_2$ in children at a PCO_2 of 40 mm Hg is 3.2 ml/100 g per minute [1]. In children with severe head injury the $CMRO_2$ is initially (12–24 h after injury) within the normal range [46] or globally decreased [48]. If the $CMRO_2$ is initially normal it falls significantly between the first and third days after injury. If the $CMRO_2$ is initially decreased it does not change significantly within this period of time. It is believed that $CMRO_2$ is decreased because of the lower metabolic activity associated with coma.

Mean $CMRO_2$ in the first 24 h is significantly higher in children with a good or moderate outcome compared to children with a poor outcome [46]. After 24 h there is no difference in $CMRO_2$ found anymore between these two groups of patients.

In children who survive $CMRO_2$ as well as $AVDO_2$ tend to rise toward the end of the period of intensive care to normal levels [46]. In children with an initial GCS of 3 or 4 the fall in $CMRO_2$ as well as the fall in $AVDO_2$ is less significant but these patients tend to present with very depressed numbers on the first measurement already.

Alternate hypothesis state that $CMRO_2$ does not accurately reflect brain metabolic demand and that ischemia could occur despite adequate supply of oxygen to the brain. Following this theory cerebral trauma might lead to mitochondrial dysfunction, preventing oxygen being utilized for aerobic metabolism [20].

Intracranial Pressure

Normal intracranial pressure (ICP) in teenagers is in the range of 10 – 15 mm Hg, normal ICP in infants is expected to be lower than 10 mm Hg. Uncontrolled increase in ICP is associated with increased mortality [4, 13, 18].

The typical finding on CAT scan correlated with increased ICP is diffuse brain swelling.

ICU treatment is directed toward keeping the ICP lower than a critical level of 15 – 20 mm Hg.

Pathologically high brain tissue pressure causes impairment of CBF and decease in venous blood flow, which lead to additional secondary brain injury [37]. Raised ICP seems to be associated with low, rather than increased CBF [27, 48]. This does not support the theory that diffuse cerebral swelling occurs as a result of excessive increase in CBF in children with head injury [9].

Increase in ICP goes parallel to an increase in brain elastance. Elastance is the ratio of change in intracranial pressure to change in intracranial volume. If the ICP is getting higher the amount of fluid volume that must be added to or subtracted from the intracranial space to make significant changes in the intracranial pressure is getting smaler and smaler. If we consider that about one third of the compliance of the CSF system is contributed to the spinal axis there might be an explanation for the fact that a lumbar drain in addition to a ventricular drain leads to significant fall in the ICP.

ICP and CBF

Several studies have emphasized the association between high ICP and hyperemia [6, 9, 17].

No significant positive correlation at the time of measurement was found between ICP and CBF in two recent studies on children with severe head injury [27, 46]. It must be considered that patients were hyperventilated at the time of CBF and ICP measurements and that different adjustments to the PCO_2 were done in the different studies. Another problem is the relation between CBF and cerebral blood volume (CBV). The CBV as one compartment of the intracranial volume might be more contributing to an increased ICP than the CBF. The other intracranial compartments are CSF, brain and extra cellular edema fluid.

Autoregulation

Autoregulation remains intact in about 60 % of head-injured children [28, 47]. Indicator for preservation of autoregulation is the significant correlation between CPP and Cerebral Vascular Resistance (CVR) [47]. This correlation is absent in the most severely injured patients. CVR is calculated from the equation CVR = CPP/CBF. Autoregulation is more impaired if the CBF is below or above two standard deviations of normal [28]. In cases with intact autoregulation mean ICP decreases with higher blood pressure and increases with lower blood pressure [28]. The cerebral venous lactate concentration seems not to be an independent determinant of CVR [47]. This speaks against the concept of vasospastic paralysis due to high levels of brain lactic acid [2, 9].

Management of Intracranial Hypertension in Pediatric Head Injury

In severely head injured children we recommend early aggressive surgical treatment for mass lesions. There are several standard therapeutic approaches for treatment of intracranial hypertension.

Elevation of the Head

Keeping the head at midline and elevation of the head up to 30 degrees supports venous return and decreases ICP. Elevation of the head also decreases CPP [22]. Adequate hydration and maintainance of MAP is required in head elevation.

Sedatives, Analgetics and Muscle Relaxants

Sedatives, analgetics and muscle relaxants control agitation, prevent increase in ICP due to stimuli such as suctioning on the tracheal tube and adapt the patient to respiratory treatment. Disadvantage of sedation is the lowering of blood pressure and impairment of neurological examination.

Antiepileptics

Some 10 % – 20 % of children with severe head injury develop seizures and require appropriate treatment with thiopental or phenytoin. Most children with posttraumatic epilepsy experience onset of seizures within the first 24 h after the injury. About 25 % of children who have early seizures may have several recurrences [41]. The prophylactic use of anticonvulsants is recommended in all children with a GCS lower than 9, in children with diffuse cerebral edema on CT scan, in patients with acute subdural hematoma and in all cases of open depressed skull fracture with parenchymal damage [23].

Intravenous Fluids

Intravenous fluids should have a normal or high sodium concentration in order to avoid hyponatremia and a fall in serum osmolality [38]. Colloidal solutions should be given as necessary to maintain normal blood pressure. Intravascular volume expansion has been shown to improve local blood flow to ischemic brain regions which appears to be mediated mainly by decreased blood viscosity [29].

Cerebral Perfusion Pressure

Cerebral perfusion pressure (CPP) needs to be maintained higher than 70 mm Hg in adolescents and teenagers and higher than 50 mm Hg in infants [10, 36, 41, 49]. CPP is determined by the Mean Arterial Pressure (MAP) and the ICP in the following way: CPP = MAP − ICP. If iv. fluids alone are not sufficient in maintaining adequate CPP phenylephrine or dopamine should be started.

Hyperventilation

Hyperventilation leads to decrease in arterial pCO_2 with a subsequent lowering of interstitial concentration of hydrogen ions and increase in tissue pH. These changes are followed by vasoconstriction of the arterioles which results in a decrease in CBF, CBV and ICP. Hyperventilation treatment must be adapted to the individual conditions of every single patient and should be based on the current values of ICP, arterial PCO_2 and $AVDO_2$ [42].

Hyperventilation in Patients with a Narrow $AVDO_2$

In head injured children the CBF is increasing to hyperemia by the first to third posttraumatic day [27, 48]. $CMRO_2$ is decreasing or staying low in the same period of time. This pattern is consistent with progressive uncoupling of CBF and metabolic demand in the sense of hyperemia or luxury perfusion. The narrow $AVDO_2$ ($AVDO_2 = CMRO_2/CBF$) is an indicator for this process [48]. The positive correlation between a low $AVDO_2$, parallel to hyperemia and a low GCS is indicative of more significant uncoupling of CBF and metabolism at deeper levels of coma [27] Hyperventilation to decrease CBF might be beneficial in these patients. The PCO_2 should not be lower than 30 mm Hg. A widening $AVDO_2$ would be an indicator for the critical reduction of CBF compared to the metabolic demand.

The greatest relative reduction in ICP seems to occur when the PCO_2 is lowered from normal to 35 mm Hg [18]. Animal studies have shown that if hyperventilation is prolonged beyond 6 h, CBF returns to normal despite the fact that the PCO_2 is still low [26]. Therefore hyperventilation should be used only during actual ICP elevations.

If CBF and $CMRO_2$ are both increased coupling between oxygen demand and perfusion would be considered.

Hyperventilation in Patients with a Wide AVDO$_2$

In the situation of decreased CBF and increased CMRO$_2$ uncoupling between blood flow and metabolic demand in the sense of ischemia must be considered. A widening AVDO$_2$ would be an indicator for this pattern (AVDO$_2$ = CMRO$_2$/CBF). Hyperventilation with further decrease in CBF might be dangerous for these patients, especially within the first 6 h after injury [31, 34]. CBF in brain contusions is significantly reduced relative to surrounding brain parenchyma and PCO$_2$ vasoresposivity is usually present. These lesions are particularly vulnerable to secondary injury that might be caused by uncontrolled hyperventilation [45, 50].

If CBF and CMRO$_2$ are both decreased coupling between oxygen demand and perfusion would be considered.

Mannitol

Mannitol, given at a iv. dose of 0.2–1.0 g/kg increases the osmotic gradient between brain and extracellular space and therefore has a dehydrating effect. Mannitol administration also reduces blood viscosity. Mannitol requires ICP monitoring to prevent rare inverse reactions by penetrating through a disrupted blood brain barrier. Serum osmolality, electrolytes and Central Venous Pressure (CVP) need to be monitored closely. Mannitol should be hold at a serum osmolality of about 310 and in case of hypotension or hemodynamic instability. Mannitol and furosemide when used together lead to a more significant and longer lasting decrease in ICP than mannitol alone [16].

Barbiturates

Application of pentobarbital is a treatment option when other methods have failed and the ICP is still persisting high. Barbiturate coma requires continuous EEG-monitoring. The maximum in therapeutic brain activity suppression is reached when the EEG shows burst suppression patterns. The suppression isoelectric EEG reading should not last longer than 10–15 s alternating with burst activity of 3–5 s.

It might be the fact that only patients with a good prognosis per se respond to barbiturate treatment with lowering of ICP while patients with a poor prognosis do not respond [24]. The prophylactic use of pentobarbital coma does not improve the outcome of adult head-injured patients [19]. Side effects such as significant reduction of MAP, cardiovascular depression associated with arrhythmias and also oliguria were observed after administration of pentobarbital in children [16, 24].

Decompressive Craniectomy

Decompressive craniectomy after head injury is only applicable to a very selected number of pediatric patients and is one of the last steps in the management of head injury. Recommended criteria for the craniectomy are initial GCS between 4 and 8, CPP lower than 60 mm Hg, uncontrolled ICP with values higher than 45 mm Hg, absence of diastolic with presence of systolic flow pattern on TCD. CT scan is necessary to rule out a mass lesion that could be responsible for the uncontrolled ICP [44].

The discussed mechanism by which the ICP was controlled in the reported patients was, that removal of the skull resulted in improved venous drainage.

Controversies

Steroids have no significant positive effect on posttraumatic brain edema, neurological status, ICP or outcome in human brain injury [6, 12, 21].

Controlled Lumbar Drainage

Ventriculostomy is considered to be one of the first and most important surgical options of treatment for increased ICP. Beside of the need for a pressure monitor the draining of CSF is essential for lowering the pressure by removing fluid. Controlled lumbar drainage of CSF in addition to ventricular drainage must be considered a new therapeutic approach in pediatric patients with manifested high ICP when all other used methods had been ineffective [30, 43].

Application of a lumbar drain is a technique that results in rapid control of intracranial hypertension.

Among the reported patients the initial ICP readings were between 25 and 50 mm Hg and the ICP four hours after drain placement was between 10 and 22 mm Hg. Lumbar drain placement was not responsible for herniation in any of these patients [43]. The drainage height of the lumbar drain should be set equal with the ventriculostomy to prevent a pressure gradient.

In severe head injury associated with extra cellular brain edema, hyperemia and decreased CSF outflow the increase in ICP is contributed to an pressure increase in all intracranial compartments. The typical CAT scan shows diffuse brain swelling and small ventricles. These findings are similar to patterns seen in pseudotumor cerebri. An external lumbar drain provides the spinal axis up to the basal cisterns with CSF drainage in addition to the drainage that is obtained from the ventriculostomy. In the situation of elevated intracranial elastance this additional drainage of CSF leads to a significant decrease within the pressure of the CSF compartment and in ICP.

Lumbar drain placement is recommended in patients in which focal mass lesion is excluded or removed and open basal cisterns are found on CT scan. In all patients a ventricular drain should be in place.

Summary

Severely head injured children present with a low global CBF in the early hours postinjury and develop hyperemia within 1–3 days. $AVDO_2$ and $CMRO_2$ tend to fall significantly within the same period of time. Autoregulation is often preserved but may be impaired in the most severely injured patients.

In severely head injured children we recommend frequent repeat CT scans as needed, early aggressive surgical treatment for mass lesions, placement of ventricular drain if safely possible and monitoring of ICP. Patients management requires early protection of the airways and hyperventilation. Hyperventilation regimen should be based on the monitored PCO_2 and $AVDO_2$ values. The PCO_2 should not be lower than 30 mm Hg. Patients with uncoupling between high CBF and low metabolic demand, indicated by a narrow $AVDO_2$, might benefit from hyperventilation. Uncontrolled hyperventilation in patients with a low CBF and a wide $AVDO_2$ has the potential risk of causing ischemia, especially on the first day postinjury. We recommend the controlled use of Mannitol in combination with furosemide. The use of barbiturates remains controversy and might be considered in some patients. The selective use of a lumbar drain appears promising for control of increased ICP when all other used methods had been ineffective.

References

1. Kennedy C, Sokoloff L (1957) An adaption of the nitrous oxide method to the study of the cerebral circulation in children; normal values for cerebral blood flow and cerebral metabolic rate in childhood. J Clin Invest 36: 1130–1137
2. Lassen NA (1966) The luxury perfusion syndrome and its possible relation to acute metabolic acidosis localized within the brain. Lancet 11: 1113–1115
3. Overgaard J, Tweed WA (1974) Cerebral circulation after head injury. Part 1: Cerebral blood flow and its regulation after closed head injury with emphasis on clinical correlations. J Neurosurg 41: 531–541
4. Miller JD, Becker DP, Ward JD, Sullivan HG, Adams WE, Rosner MJ (1977) Significance of intracranial hypertension in severe head injury. J Neurosurg 47: 503–516
5. Bruce DA, Raphaely RC, Goldberg AI, Zimmerman RA, Bilaniuk LT, Schut L, Kuhl DE (1979) Pathophysiology, treatment and outcome following severe head injury in children. Childs brain 5: 174–191
6. Cooper PR, Moody S, Clark WK, Kirkpatrick J, Marvilla K, Gould AL, Drane W (1979) Dexamethasone and severe head injury. A prospective double blind study. J Neurosurg 51: 307–316
7. Obrist WD, Gennarelli TA, Segawa H, Dolinskas CA, Langfitt TW (1979) Relation of cerebral blood flow to neurological status and outcome in head injured patients. J Neurosurg 51: 292–300
8. Settergren G, Lindblad BS, Persson B (1980) Cerebral blood flow and exchange of oxygen, glucose ketone bodies, lactate, pyruvate and amino acids in anesthetized children. Acta Paediatr Scand 69: 457–465
9. Bruce DA, Alavi A, Bilaniuk L, Dolinskas C, Obrist W, Uzzell B (1981) Diffuse cerebral swelling following head injuries in children: the syndrome of "malignant brain edema." J Neurosurg 54: 170–178
10. Miller JD, Butterworth JF, Gudeman SK, Faulkner JE, Choi SC, Selhorst JB, Harbison JW, Lutz HA, Young HF, Becker DP (1981) Further experience in the management of severe head injury. J Neurosurg 54: 289–299

11. Overgaard J, Mosdal C, Tweed WA (1981) Cerebral circulation after head injury. III. Does reduced regional cerebral blood flow determine recovery of brain function after blunt head injury? J Neurosurg 55: 63–74
12. Saul TG, Ducker TB, Salcman M, Carro E (1981) Steroids in severe head injury: a prospective randomized clinical trial. J Neurosurg 54: 596–600
13. Saul TG, Ducker TB (1982) Effect of intracranial pressure monitoring and aggressive treatment on mortality in severe head injury. J Neurosurg 56: 498–503
14. Younkin DP, Reivich M, Jaggi J, Obrist W, Delivoria-Papadopoulos M (1982) Noninvasive method of estimating human newborn regional cerebral blood flow. J Cereb Blood Flow Metab 2: 415–420
15. Pollay M, Fullenwider C, Roberts PA, Stevens FA (1983) Effect of mannitol and furosemide on blood brain osmotic gradient and intracranial pressure. J Neurosurg 59: 945–950
16. Traeger SM, Henning RJ, Dobkin W, Giannotta S, Weil MH, Weiss M (1983) Hemodynamic effects of pentobarbital therapy for intracranial hypertension. Crit Care Med 11: 697–701
17. Obrist WD, Langfitt TW, Jaggi JL, Cruz J, Gennarelli TA (1984) Cerebral blood flow and metabolism in comatose patients with acute head injury. Relationship to intracranial hypertension. J Neurosurg 61: 241–253
18. Berger MS, Pitts LH, Lovely M, Edwards MS, Bartkowski HM (1985) Outcome from severe head injury in children and adolescents. J Neurosurg 62: 194–199
19. Ward JD, Becker DP, Miller JD, Choi SC, Marmarou A, Wood C, Newlon PG, Keenan R (1985) Failure of prophylactic barbiturate coma in the treatment of severe head injury. J Neurosurg 62: 383–388
20. Yang MS, DeWitt DS, Becker DP, Hayes RL (1985) Regional brain metabolite levels following mild experimental head injury in the cat. J Neurosurg 63: 617–621
21. Dearden NM, Gibson JS, McDowall DG, Gibson RM, Cameron MM (1986) Effect of high dose dexamethasone on outcome from severe head injury. J Neurosurg 64: 81–88
22. Rosner MJ, Coley IB (1986) Cerebral perfusion pressure, intracranial pressure and head elevation. J Neurosurg 65: 636–641
23. Hahn YS, Fuchs S, Flannary AM, Barthel MJ, McLone DG (1988) Factors influencing post-traumatic seizures in children. Neurosurgery 22: 864–867
24. Kasoff SS, Lansen TA, Holder D, Filippo JS (1988) Aggressive physiologic monitoring of pediatric head trauma patients with elevated intracranial pressure. Pediatr Neuroscience 14: 241–249
25. Luerssen TG, Klauber MR, Marshall LF (1988) Outcome from head injury related to patients age. J Neurosurg 68: 409–416
26. Muizelaar JP, van der Poel HG, Li ZC, Kontos HA, Lavasseur JE (1988) Pial arteriolar vessel diameter and CO_2 reactivity during prolonged hyperventilation in the rabbit. J Neurosurg 69: 923–927
27. Muizelaar JP, Marmarou A, DeSalles AA, Ward JD, Zimmermann RS, Li Z, Choi SC, Young HF (1989) Cerebral blood flow and metabolism in severely head injured chidren. I. Relationship between GSC score, outcome, ICP and PVI. J Neurosurg 71: 63–71
28. Muizelaar JP, Ward JD, Marmarou A, Newlon PG, Wachi A (1989) Cerebral blood flow and metabolism in severely head injured children. I. Autoregulation. J Neurosurg 71: 72–76
29. Bouma GJ, Muizelaar JP (1990) Relationship between cardiac output and cerebral blood flow in patients with intact and with impaired autoregulation. J Neurosurg 73: 368–374
30. Baldwin HZ, Rekate HL (1991) Preliminary experience with controlled external lumbar drainage in diffuse pediatric head injury. Pediatr Neurosurg 17: 115–120
31. Bouma GJ, Muizelaar JP, Choi SC, Newlon PG, Young HF (1991) Cerebral circulation and metabolism after severe traumatic brain injury: the elusive role of ischemia. J Neurosurg 75: 685–693
32. Marion DW, Derby J, Yonas H (1991) Acute regional cerebral blood flow changes caused by severe head injuries. J Neurosurg 74: 407–414
33. Luerssen TG (1991) Head injuries in children. Neurosurg Clin North Am 2: 399–410
34. Muizelaar JP, Marmarou A, Ward JD, Kontos HA, Choi SC, Becker DP, Gruemer H, Young HF (1991) Adverse effects of prolonged hyperventilation in patients with severe head injury: a randomized clinical trial. J Neurosurg 75: 731–739
35. Sharples PM, Stuart AG, Aynsley-Green A, Heaviside D, Pay DA, McGann A, Crawford PJ,

Harpin R, Eyre JA (1991) A practical method of serial bedside measurement of cerebral blood flow and metabolism during neurointensive care. Arch Dis Child 66: 1326–1332

36. Chan KH, Dearden NM, Miller JD, Andrews PJ, Midgley S (1993) Multimodality monitoring as a guide to treatment of intracranial hypertension after severe brain injury. Neurosurgery 32: 547–553
37. Miller JD, Piper IR, Dearden NM (1993) Management and intracranial hypertension in head injury: matching treatment with cause. Acta Neurochir Suppl 57: 152–159
38. Pfenninger J (1993) Neurological intensive care in children. Intenisive Care Med 19: 243–250
39. Alexander MJ, Martin NA, Khanna R, Caron M, Becker DP (1994) Regional cerebral blood flow trends in head injured patients with focal contusions and cerebral edema. Acta Neurochir Suppl 60: 479–481
40. Lang DA, Teasdale GT, Macpherson P, Lawrence A (1994) Diffuse brain swelling after head injury: more often malignant in adults than in children? J Neurosurg 80: 675–680
41. Goldstein B, Powers KS (1994) Head trauma in children. Pediatr Rev 6: 213–219
42. Miller JD (1994) Swelling and blood flow in the injured child's brain. Lancet 344: 421–422
43. Levy DL, Rekate HL, Cherny WB, Manwaring KH, Moss SD, Baldwin HZ (1995) Controlled lumbar drain in pediatric head injury. J Neurosurg 83: 453–460
44. Morgalla MH, Krasznai L, Buchholz R, Bitzer M, Deusch H, Walz G-U, Grote EH (1995) Repeated decompressive craniectomy after head injury in children: two successful cases as result of improved neuromonitoring. Surg Neurol 43: 583–590
45. Schroeder ML, Muizelaar JP, Bullock MS, Salvant JB, Povlishok JT (1995) Focal ischemia due to traumatic contusions documented by stable xenon CT and ultrastructural studies. J Neurosurg 82: 966–971
46. Sharples PM, Stuart AG, Matthews DSF, Aynsley-Green A, Eyre JA (1995) Cerebral blood flow and metabolism in children with severe head injury. I. Relation to age, Glasgow coma score, outcome, intracranial pressure and time after injury. J Neurol Neurosurg Psychiatry 58: 145–152
47. Sharples PM, Matthews DSF, Eyre JA (1995) Cerebral blood flow and metabolism in children with severe head injuries. II. cerebrovascular resistance and its determinants. J Neurol Neurosurg Psychiatry 58: 153–159
48. Beyda DH (1996) Time course of cerebral blood flow and metabolism in pediatric head trauma. 25th Educational and Scientific Symposium, Society of Critical Care Medicine, 5–9 February
49. Giulioni M, Ursino M (1996) Impact of cerebral perfusion pressure and autoregulation on intracranial dynamics: a modeling study. Neurosurg 39: 1005–1015
50. McLaughlin MR, Marion DW (1996) Cerebral blood flow and vasoresponsivity within and around cerebral contusions. J Neurosurg 85: 871–876

12 Quality and Therapeutic Advances in Multimodality Neuromonitoring Following Head Injury

J. Meixensberger, A. Jäger, J. Dings, S. Baunach, and K. Roosen

Introduction

While primary brain damage after trauma cannot be influenced by therapy, the major goal in the treatment of severely head injured patients is to prevent secondary ischemic brain damage. It is well known that secondary ischemic insults caused by arterial hypoxia and hypocapnia, systemic hypotension, or increased intracranial pressure (ICP) destroy functional brain tissue and worsen outcome after acute brain injury [2].

The importance of acute hemodynamic disturbances and the variability of cerebral blood flow following head injury is well documented by noncontinuously performed cerebral blood flow (CBF) measurements (133xenon, stable xenon) [1, 9, 12, 14]. Therefore in clinical routine the best technique to detect hemodynamic changes and ischemic episodes is sensitive, continuous monitoring of CBF and cerebral oxygenation. It should supplement standard neuromonitoring including ICP, mean arterial pressure (MAP), and cerebral perfusion pressure (CPP). This is especially important because CPP can give us only an estimation of global cerebral perfusion. The critical level of CPP is below 70 mm Hg. However, a comparative analysis between CPP and CBF revealed that a CPP above 70 mm Hg guarantees not in every case a sufficient cerebral perfusion [12].

Nowadays there are different sensitive hemodynamic continuous monitoring methods applicable in the intensive care unit.

The jugular venous oximetry [15] is an invasive global/hemispheric method which determines cerebral oxygenation only indirectly. Brain tissue pO_2 [$p(ti)O_2$] measurement [4, 5, 7, 13, 16] is an invasive, regional method. $p(ti)O_2$ reflects the balance between the oxygen offer and the oxygen consumption of the brain tissue. It depends on the arterial oxygen and carbon dioxide pressure, MAP, ICP, CPP and cellular metabolism, cerebral blood flow, and especially the state of the cerebral microcirculation. Regional oxygen saturation (rSO_2) using near infrared spectroscopy [8, 10] is a noninvasive technique. The calculation of regional cerebral oxygenation within the microvasculature of the brain is based on spectroscopic data from multiple wavelengths of oxygenated and desoxygenated hemoglobin collected by two detectors, distinguishing between shallow and deep tissue oxygenation.

The goal of our study was to check the quality of these new hemodynamic monitoring techniques. Additionally, we analyzed the time course of ischemic insults and consequences for targeted treatment of raised ICP taking cerebral hemodynamics under consideration.

Patients and Methods

A total of 45 severely head injured patients (GCS $\leq$ 8, age 31.3 $\pm$ 9.8 years) with diffuse (n = 28) or focal brain injury (n = 17) were studied an average of 7.5 $\pm$ 3.4 days (range 1 – 16) on the neurosurgical ICU. All patients were treated using a standard therapeutic protocol that emphasized immediate evacuation of space-occupying intracranial hematomas. They were treated to control ICP below 20 mm Hg and CPP above 70 mm Hg. ICP greater than 20 mm Hg was treated by sedation (combination of midazolam and fentanyl), moderate hyperventilation (paCO$_2$ 30 – 35 mm Hg) and intravenous administration of mannitol and/or glycerol. Barbiturate coma started if ICP was refractory to the above treatment. Finally, THAM (Tris) buffer was coadministered and, if raised ICP was uncontrollable, decompressive craniectomy was performed. Volume expansion and vasopressors were given in case of CPP < 70 mm Hg caused by arterial hypotension. Arterial paO$_2$, paCO$_2$, pH, BE were determined to control systemic oxygenation, and body temperature was measured continuously.

Permission to perform multimodal neuromonitoring was given by the local ethics committee. Neuromonitoring included ICP (Camino Laboratories, San Diego, USA), MAP, recorded from a radial arterial catheter calibrated to the Foramen of Monroi (Exadyn Combitrans device, Braun Melsungen, Melsungen, Germany), the calculated CPP (= MAP minus ICP), endtidal CO$_2$ (CO$_2$et; Dräger-Werk, Lübeck, Germany), regional brain p(ti)O$_2$(LICOX System, GMS, Kiel-Mielkendorf, Germany), rSO$_2$INVOS 3100 Oximeter, Somanetics, Detroit, USA), and S$_j$O$_2$ (Oximetrix-3 System, Abbott Laboratories, North Chicago, USA). The brain p(ti)O$_2$ catheter was usually inserted in addition to the tissue ICP probe in CT-visible normal brain (white matter). The side of insertion was routinely on the right frontal side if there was a diffuse brain injury, or on the affected side if there was a hemispheric or focal lesion. The insertion technique is described elsewhere in detail [4, 5].

Transcranial cerebral oximetry was performed attaching the disposable sensor pad to the patients frontal skin at the same side of ICP, p(ti)O$_2$ monitoring [10]. The S$_j$O$_2$ monitoring was performed after placement of a fiberoptic catheter into the the jugular bulb corresponding to the technique described by Robertson et al. [15]. Data sampling and storage (every 10 s) in ASCII data files were carried out using a personal computer (Intel 486/75 Mhz, 16 AD converter, 16 Mbyte RAM, 1 Gbyte hard disk; Neutec-Computer, von Zeppelin, Pullach, Germany) working on a MS-DOS/windows program. After detecting and eliminating artifacts (by several independent physicians according to a clinical protocol) data were statistically evaluated with a self-developed program based on Mathematica running on an UNIX workstation to handle large data files (500 kByte per day of monitoring). Only nonparametric statistical methods were used. All results were displayed graphically. Time of good data quality was calculated by the formula: time of good data quality (%) = 100 – (time of artifacts (min)×100)/total monitoring time (min).

Multimodal Hemodynamic Neuromonitoring

Safety and Data Quality

Table 1 summarizes data concerning reliability and data quality of the three hemodynamic monitoring techniques. Invasive $p(ti)O_2$ monitoring so far caused no infection by the catheter for a mean monitoring time of 7 days. In two cases (2.7 %) a small, non-space-occupying hematoma was seen (n = 70) [5]. No evacuation was necessary. Mean sensitivity drift of the catheter was < 10 %, and zero drift was 1.5 ± 1.5 mm Hg [4, 5]. Good data quality was calculated up to 95 %. Sensitivity to changes of cerebral hemodynamics (CPP, S_jO_2, blood flow velocity) has been demonstrated by various studies [4, 7, 16]. While rSO_2 using near infrared spectroscopy allows detection of hemodynamic changes under certain circumstances [8, 10], analysis of our long-term monitoring over time after acute brain injury (2425 h) revealed a good data reading of only up to 70 %. In operated patients often a transcranial measurement of rSO_2 is impossible due to subdural air or a galea hematoma. In addition to reliability, sensitivity of rSO_2 was also restricted compared to both $p(ti)O_2$ and S_jO_2. Comparative measurements of S_jO_2 were performed only in selected cases (n = 5). However, our observations concerning difficulties during S_jO_2 monitoring agreed with other reports [7, 16] about the limited reliability. Good data quality during long-term monitoring only reached 40 % – 50 % [7].

As a consequence of practicability and reliability we analyzed in our clinical set up the validity of $p(ti)O_2$ as an example of an additional hemodynamic monitoring technology.

Table 1. Quality of multimodal hemodynamic neuromonitoring: brain tissue – pO_2 [$p(ti)O_2$], regional oxygen saturation (rSO_2), jugular bulb oxygen saturation (S_jO_2)

$p(ti)O_2$	Regional, invasive	Sensitive	Reliable	Good data quality: to 95%
rSO_2	Regional, noninvasive	Sensitive?	Limited reliable	Good data quality: 50% – 70% (if measurement is possible)
S_jO_2	Global, invasive	Sensitive	Limited reliable	Good data quality: 40% – 50%

Time Course of Cerebral Oxygenation After Head Injury

The time course of p(ti)O_2 was calculated from 40 head-injured patients (Fig. 1). The first 2 days after injury p(ti)O_2 generally ranged below 15 mm Hg. On days 3–5 a relative increase to hyperemic p(ti)O_2 (> 30 mm Hg) was observed, corresponding to an increase in blood flow velocity in the middle cerebral artery [4], which decreased to normal levels of p(ti)O_2 after day 6. In a second step the distribution of three different p(ti)O_2 classes (< 15 mm Hg, 15–30 mm Hg, > 30 mm Hg) were analyzed. Critical low p(ti)O_2 values (< 15 mm Hg) were observed in more than 50 % on day 1 and in approximately 25 % on day 2. A second peak was found after day 6. This characteristic distribution fits well with the time course of CPP insults reported by Cortbus et al. [2]. Ad-

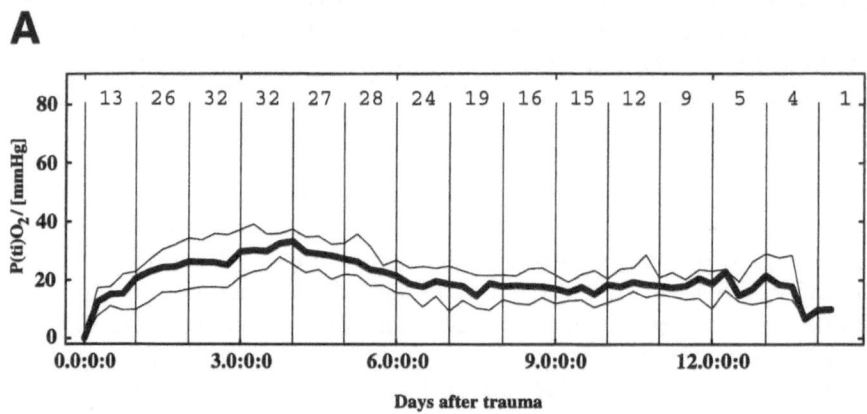

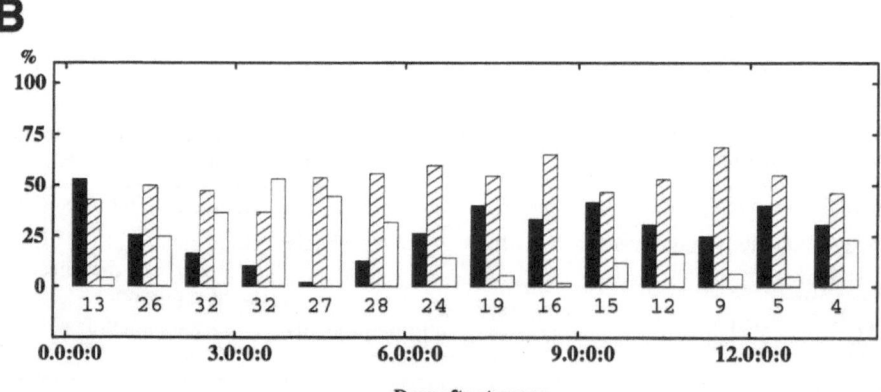

Fig. 1A,B. Time course of brain tissue pO_2 [p(ti)O_2 after severe head injury; n = 40 patients]. Graphs were calculated from ASCII data files of 40 patients after eliminating artifacts by several independant physicians. **A** Median p(ti)O_2(standard deviation every 6 h. Top line, number of patients included per day after trauma. **B** Corresponding histogram distribution [< 15 mm Hg (black column), 15–30 mm Hg (hatched column), > 30 mm Hg (white column)] of p(ti)O_2. Bottom line, number of included patients per day after trauma

ditionally, critical p(ti)O$_2$ values demonstrated the importance of early ischemia after trauma, in agreement with findings of CBF measurements [1, 9].
Most ischemic p(ti)O$_2$ episodes were caused by raised ICP, systemic hypotension, hypocapnia, and, rarely, systemic hypoxia.

Effect of Therapy on Cerebral Oxygenation

Effect of Induced Hypertension

Systemic hypotension is one of the major factors worsening secondary ischemic brain damage. Figure 2 illustrates the effect of decrease and therapeutic
increase in MAP on cerebral oxygenation [p(ti)O$_2$ and rSO$_2$] over time after
acute head injury. In contrast to others [7], at a CPP level of 70 mm Hg we
found critical low brain p(ti)O$_2$ (7 mm Hg), which was normalized increasing
MAP and CPP. On the other hand, normal p(ti)O$_2$ was detected at decreased
CPP (< 70 mm Hg) These findings confirm earlier comparative CBF/CPP studies indicating individual and time-dependent variation in critical CPP borders [12]. In our experience, on-line monitoring of p(ti)O$_2$ enables the deter-
mination of sufficient CPP from patient to patient and from day to day.

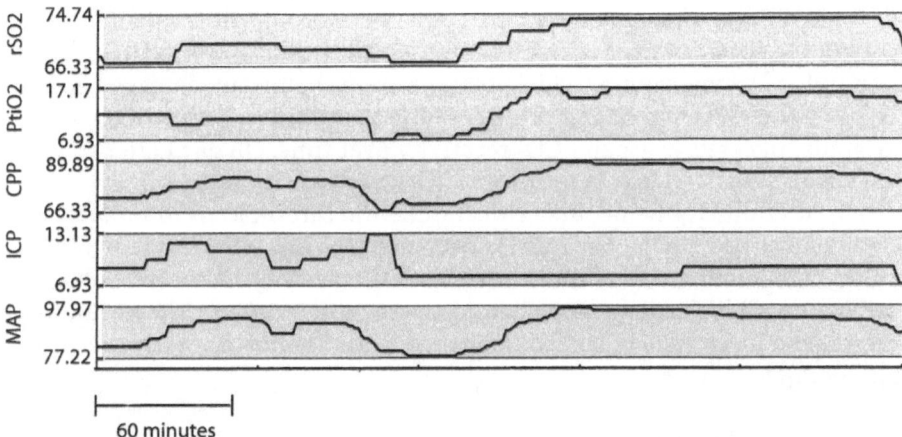

Fig. 2. Multimodal hemodynamic neuromonitoring. MAP, Mean arterial pressure (mm Hg);
ICP, intracranial pressure (mm Hg); CPP, cerebral perfusion pressure (mm Hg); p(ti)O$_2$, regional brain tissue pO$_2$ (mm Hg); rSO$_2$, regional oxygen saturation (%). The effect of induced
hypertension was monitored and balanced on-line. A marked decline in MAP to 77 mm Hg
(arrow) induced a decrease in CPP to around 70 mm Hg and a critical p(ti)O$_2$ (7 mm Hg). After
elevation of MAP (100 mm Hg) critical p(ti)O$_2$ increased to values around 17 mm Hg. The
simultaneous time course of rSO$_2$ was monitored using near infrared spectroscopy. Normal
ICP was not affected by induced hypertension, indicating intact autoregulation

Effect of Induced Hypocapnia (Hyperventilation Therapy)

Induced hypocapnia is one of the main therapeutic tools in the treatment of intracranial hypertension: the reduction of ICP is added to a decrease in cerebral blood volume after vasoconstriction of pial vessels and arterioles. The risk of inducing ischemia depends on the baseline level of CBF and on intact or disturbed cerebrovascular CO_2 reactivity [3, 11]. Analyzing 80 measurements (performed in 24 patients) after induced hypocapnia (baseline $paCO_2$ 33.4 ± 1.4 mm Hg decreased to 26.6 ± 1.3 mm Hg) on days 0–9 after trauma, we distinguished between a group with a $p(ti)O_2$ values less than 15 and one with values greater than 15 mm Hg. Patients with a critical low $p(ti)O_2$ (< 15 mm Hg) may be at higher risk of ischemic brain damage. In 30 % of our cases we found a baseline $p(ti)O_2$ below 15 mm Hg. In most cases we found low $p(ti)O_2$ values in the first days after brain injury and a second peak after day 6 (Fig. 1). In 70 % of our cases $p(ti)O_2$ was above 15 mm Hg. There was no significant difference in $paCO_2$, paO_2, CPP, or age between the two groups. Taking in consideration the absolute level of $p(ti)O_2$, we analyzed the risk of inducing an ischemic $p(ti)O_2$ level with induced hypocapnia combined with an intact cerebrovascular CO_2 reactivity, which we found in 75 % of our cases [6]. In the group with a $p(ti)O_2$ above 15 mm Hg the resting $p(ti)O_2$ decreased at an average from 29 to 24 mm Hg, never approaching the ischemic threshold of 10 mm Hg after decrease in $paCO_2$. Only in the group with a $p(ti)O_2$ below 15 mm Hg – about 26 % of our cases – we did find critical low $p(ti)O_2$ values after induced hypocapnia, which may cause ischemia in damaged brain. Figure 3 should clarify the importance of the absolute level of $p(ti)O_2$ and the variability of cerebrovascular CO_2 reactivity over time. On day 1 after trauma the change in $paCO_2$ from 34 to 28 mm Hg induced a critical drop in initial low $p(ti)O_2$ of 12 mm Hg below the critical ischemic threshold of 10 mm Hg. On day 4 the resting $p(ti)O_2$ of 28 mm Hg decreased to about 18 after changing the $paCO_2$, indicating an increase in $p(ti)O_2$ CO_2 reactivity. However, values of $p(ti)O_2$, possibly leading to ischemia, were not induced. These findings recommend a carefully balanced indication and monitoring of hyperventilation therapy.

Effect of Osmodiuretics (Mannitol)

Mannitol is an effective drug for reducing ICP and thus improving CPP. Analyzing 28 studies (performed in 11 patients) after administration of mannitol (0.5 g/kg body weight), we distinguished three groups based on the initial $p(ti)O_2$: < 15 mm Hg, 15–30 mm Hg, and > 30 mm Hg. While in all three groups a similiar significant decrease in ICP and increase in CPP could be detected after mannitol, the effect on $p(ti)O_2$ differed between the different groups: in the group with reduced $p(ti)O_2$ (< 15 mm Hg; $n = 6$) there was an improvement in $p(ti)O_2$ (> 1 0 % increase) in four cases and no change in two; in the second group: $p(ti)O_2$ 15–30 mm Hg (n = 12) in six cases $p(ti)O_2$ improved and in six no change or a decrease in microcirculation could be seen; in the hyperemic group: $p(ti)O_2$ > 30 mm Hg ($n = 10$) generally a decrease or no change of $p(ti)O_2$

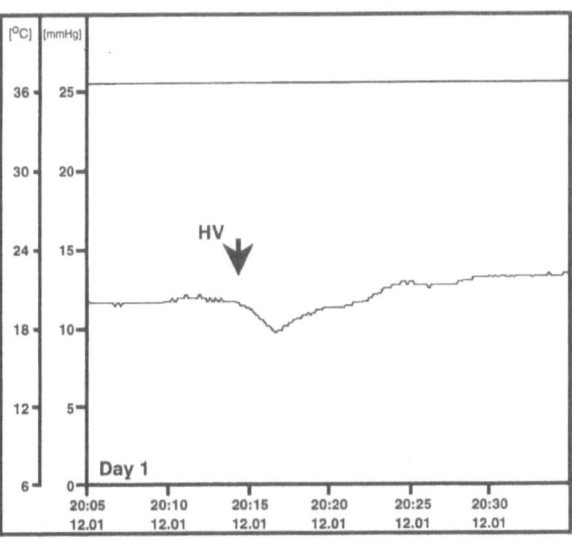

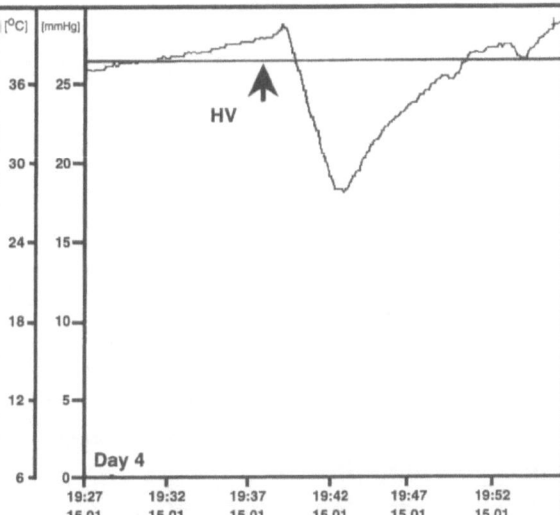

Fig. 3. Hyperventilation therapy (HV) for treatment of raised intracranial pressure, original tissue, pO_2 [p(ti)-O_2]; chart of a severely head-injured patient after change in $paCO_2$. Top, day 1 after trauma: induced hypocapnia ($paCO_2$ 28 mm Hg) decreased critical low $p(ti)O_2$ [$p(ti)O_2$ <10 – 15 mm Hg] to lower level, which normalized under baseline conditions ($paCO_2$ 34 mm Hg). Bottom, day 4 after trauma: induced hypocapnia ($paCO_2$ 27 mm Hg) decreased baseline, $p(ti)O_2$ above 25 mm Hg. However, despite intact cerebrovascular CO_2 reactivity a critical level of $p(ti)O_2$ was not reached, and $p(ti)O_2$ normalized under baseline conditions ($paCO_2$ 33 mm Hg)

($n = 8$). These preliminary data suggest that microcirculation improves after mannitol administration especially in patients with reduced or normal $p(ti)O_2$.

Figure 4 gives a flow chart for clinical diagnosis of ischemic $p(ti)O_2$ episodes and proposed targeted therapeutic management in the clinical set up of hemodynamic neuromonitoring.

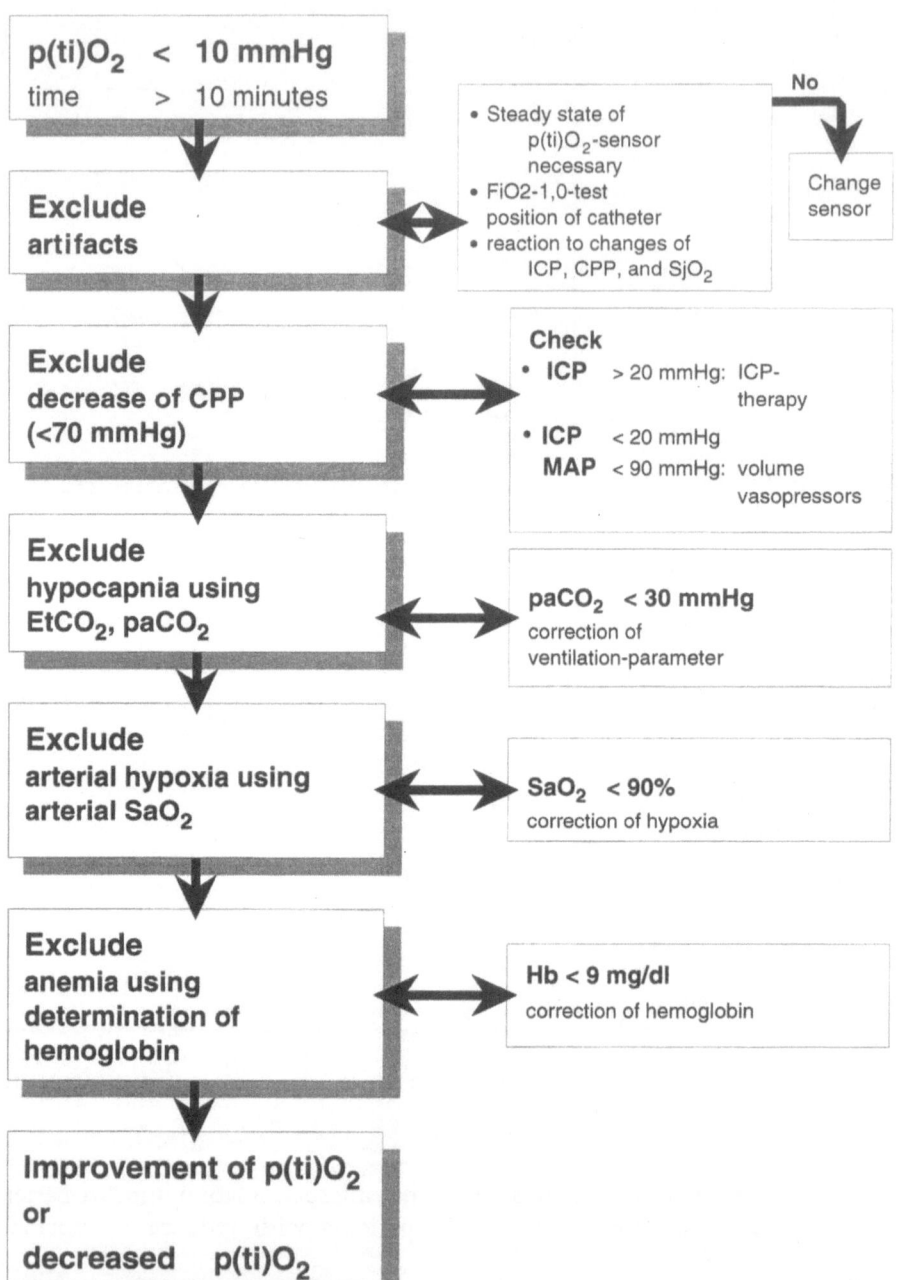

Fig. 4. Flow chart for clinical diagnosis of critical episodes of regional tissue pO_2 [$p(ti)O_2$ < 10 −15 mm Hg]

Summary and Conclusion

Multimodal monitoring of cerebral hemodynamics supplements neuromonitoring (ICP, MAP, CPP) in the treatment of severely head-injured patients. However, only regional $p(ti)O_2$ is a safe, reliable, and sensitive method for cerebral oxygenation after acute brain injury. Monitoring of $p(ti)O_2$ is superior to S_jO_2 in data quality and reliability. In clinical routine noninvasively monitoring of rSO_2 using near infrared spectroscopy is not reliable and sensitive enough to provide sufficient information about cerebral hemodynamics over the entire period after acute brain injury. Further improvements in the technique seem to be necessary. Early detection of critical episodes of regional microcirculation [$p(ti)O_2 < 10 - 15$ mm Hg] enables a targeted therapy (Fig. 4). Induced hypertension can be balanced to determine sufficient CPP. Hyperventilation therapy, especially $paCO_2$ below 30 mm Hg, is indicated only in patients with normal or hyperemic cerebral oxygenation status. In patients with reduced cerebral oxygenation mannitol administration should be first choice to treat raised ICP. Reduction of critical $p(ti)O_2$ values helps to minimize the risk of secondary ischemic brain damage. This will hopefully improve outcome of critically ill head-injured patients.

Acknowledgements. Supported by Deutsche Forschungsgemeinschaft (Me 1020/3-1).

References

1. Bouma GJ, Muizelaar JP, Stringer WA et al (1992) Ultra-early evaluation of regional cerebral blood flow in severely head-injured patients using xenon-enhanced computerized tomography. J Neurosurg 77: 360 – 368
2. Cortbus F, Jonas PA, Miller JD et al (1994) Cause, distribution and significance of episodes of reduced cerebral perfusion pressure following head injury. Acta Neurochir 130: 117 – 124
3. Darby JM, Yonas H, Marion DW et al (1988) Local "inverse steal" induced by hyper-ventilation in head injury. Neurosurgery 23: 84 – 88
4. Dings J, Meixensberger J, Amschler J et al (1996) Brain tissue pO$_2$ relation to cerebral perfusion pressure, TCD findings and TCD-CO$_2$-reactivity after severe head injury. Acta Neurochir 138: 425 – 434
5. Dings J, Meixensberger J, Roosen K (1997) Brain tissue pO$_2$-monitoring: catheter-stability and complications. Neurol Research in press
6. Dings J, Meixensberger J, Amschler J, Roosen K (1996) Continuous monitoring of brain tissue pO$_2$: a new tool to minimize the risk of ischemia caused by hyperventilation therapy. Zbl Neurochir 57: 177 – 183
7. Kiening KL, Unterberg AW, Bardt TF et al (1996) Monitoring of cerebral oxygenation in patients with severe head injuries: brain tissue pO$_2$ versus jugular rein oxygen saturation. J Neurosurg 85: 751 – 757
8. Kirkpatrick PJ, Smielewski P, Czosnyka M et al (1995) Near-infrared spectroscopy use in patients with head injury. J Neurosurg 83: 963 – 970
9. Marion DW, Darby J, Yonas H (1991) Acute regional cerebral blood flow changes caused by severe head injuries. J Neurosurg 74: 407 – 414
10. McCormick P, Stewart M, Goelting M, Dujovny M, Lewis G, Ausman JI (1991) Noninvasive cerebral optical spectroscopy for monitoring cerebral oxygen delivering and hemodynamics. Neurosurg 36(5): 1033 – 1036
11. Meixensberger J, Brawanski A, Holzschuh M, Danhauser-Leistner I, Ullrich W (1991) CBF

dynamics during hyperventilation therapy for intracranial hypertension. In: Bock WJ, Lumenta C, Brock M, Klinger M (eds) Advances of neurosurgery, vol 19. Springer, Berlin Heidelberg New York, pp 240–244

12. Meixensberger J (1993) Xenon 133-CBF measurements in severe head injury and sub-arachnoid haemorrhage. Acta Neurochir 59: 28–33
13. Meixensberger J, Dings J, Kuhnigk H, Roosen K (1993) Studies of tissue pO_2 in normal and pathological human brain cortex. Acta Neurochir [Suppl] 59: 58–63
14. Obrist WD, Langfitt TW, Jaggi JL et al (1984) Cerebral blood flow and metabolism in com-atose patients with acute head injury. J Neurosurg 61: 241–253
15. Robertson CS, Narayan RK, Gokaslan AL, Pahwa R, Grossman RG, Caram P Jr, Allen E (1989) Cerebral arteriovenous oxygen difference as an estimate of cerebral blood flow in comatose patients. J Neurosurg 70: 222–230
16. Santbrink van H, Maas AIR, Avezaat CJJ (1996) Continuous monitoring of partial pres-sure of brain tissue oxygen in patients with severe head injury. Neurosurg 38: 21–31

13 Monitoring of Cerebral Oxygenation in Traumatic Brain Injured Patients

A.S. Sarrafzadeh, A.W. Unterberg, K.L. Kiening, T.F. Bardt, G.-H. Schneider, and W.R. Lanksch

Introduction

For many years, the sequel of traumatic brain injury distinguished between primary and secondary damage. Primary damage, caused by the physical forces associated with the trauma, occurs more or less instantly and is not reversible. On the other hand, there are many occasions and opportunities for secondary or delayed brain damage to occur, even days after head injury. The most frequent causes of secondary brain damage are ischemia and hypoxia.

Ischemic brain damage is extremely common as a postmortem finding in patients with fatal head injuries [9]. It is due to a critical reduction in cerebral blood flow (< 20 ml/100 g per minute) [19] and most frequently caused by intracranial hypertension or a decrease in arterial pressure. An ischemic cerebral blood flow (CBF) has been associated with a poor neurological outcome [20] and strengthens the significance of sufficient brain perfusion. It is known that cerebral hypoperfusion can be compensated initially by means of increased extraction of oxygen, characterized by decreased CBF, elevated arteriovenous oxygen difference, $AVDO_2$ (> 3.0 mmol/ml), normal lactate, and unchanged cerebral metabolic rate of oxygen ($CMRO_2$). Ischemia occurs when further decreases in CBF cannot be compensated for by increased oxygen extraction, manifested by a fall in $CMRO_2$ and an increase in cerebral lactate production. Ischemia may end in an irreversible deficit [22]. Thus, it is most important to recognize cerebral hypoperfusion as early as possible.

Cerebral hypoxia, defined as insufficient oxygenation of brain cells, is another condition which leads to secondary brain damage with possibly irreversible consequences. It might be deleterious for the outcome of the patient if not treated in time [8]. Tissue oxygenation is the product of blood flow and arterial O_2 content perfusing the tissue over time. Thus, prevention of low CBF and hypoxemia, resulting from inadequate respiration or reduced hematocrit, is important to avoid cerebral hypoxia.

Theoretically, continuous monitoring of CBF and cerebral oxygenation is necessary to detect phases of ischemia and hypoxia. Today, the techniques for CBF measurements are time-consuming, invasive, intermittent and are not suitable for continuous monitoring of the patient. However, cerebral oxygenation can be monitored continuously. The following techniques are available and may give information about cerebral oxygenation and, indirectly, about cerebral perfusion:

1. Monitoring of cerebral tissue saturation by near-infrared spectroscopy (NIRS)
2. Jugular venous oxygen saturation monitoring ($SjvO_2$)
3. Monitoring of brain tissue oxygen pressure ($PtiO_2$)

Near-Infrared Spectroscopy (NIRS)

Near-infrared spectroscopy is a noninvasive method to monitor regional cerebral oxygenation and was first introduced for clinical application by Jobsis in 1977. It consists of a sensor fixed on the skin of the frontal area connected to a data recording device. The method is based on two facts. Firstly, in brain parenchyma there are three main chromophores, oxyhemoglobin (HbO_2), deoxyhemoglobin (HB), and oxidized cytochrome aa3 ($CytO_2$), each having a characteristic absorption spectrum for the individually transmitted wavelength. Secondly, light in the near-infrared range (700–950 nm) can pass several centimeters through biological tissue and is both scattered and absorbed, depending on the type of tissue and the amount of the different chromophores present. The NIRSsensor has one light source and several detectors measuring the amount of reflected light of the different wavelengths. This information is converted over an algorithm, integrating tissue depths, absorption properties of the skin, skull, brain, cerebrospinal fluid, and the chromophores in an oxygenation value, given as regional oxygen saturation (rSO_2) or as concentration of oxygenated/deoxygenated hemoglobin (μmol/dl) and cytochromoxydase aa3.

There is controversy in the literature about the applicability and quality of NIRS data [16, 25]. A major problem is the contribution of extracranial tissues for estimation of light path length [7]. In the majority of cases, NIRS is used as a nonquantitative method during short observation periods, e.g., in carotid endarterectomy [15]. For long-term use, as required for monitoring cerebral oxygenation in the neurointensive care unit, only a few studies have been reported and comparisons with other methods are rare. A comparison of NIRS with $SjvO_2$ revealed a significant correlation between rSO_2 (NIRS) and $SjvO_2$ during carotid endarterectomy [29], but in long-term monitoring in patients with severe head injury, NIRS was not useful clinically [16].

Monitoring of Jugular Venous Oxygen Saturation ($SjvO_2$)

Monitoring of jugular venous oxygen saturation is an already established method for continuous monitoring of cerebral oxygenation. $SjvO_2$ gives information about global cerebral oxygenation and is measured invasively. A fiberoptic catheter is placed in the internal jugular vein with the tip positioned in the jugular bulb. It is a useful clinical monitor for detecting episodes of cerebral hypoxia/ischemia or hyperemia, since $SjvO_2$ reflects the balance between oxygen delivery to the brain and oxygen consumption by the brain. Normal values are in the range of 60%–65% and may be higher in patients with severe head injury (68% ± 10%) [30]. A decrease of $SjvO_2$ below 50% is considered to indicate ischemia, above 75% hyperemia [2]. Patients with frequent episodes of decreased jugular venous oxygen saturation have a worse outcome [21]. The most common reasons for critical decreases in $SjvO_2$ are intracranial hypertension, low blood pressure, and hypocarbia. In such instances, low $SjvO_2$ can be treated by elevating the cerebral perfusion pressure and changing the respiration mode to an arterial pCO_2 between 30 – 35 mm Hg. On the other hand, if $SjvO_2$ is above 75%, indicating hyperemia, a further elevation of cerebral blood flow might be deleterious. Changes in $SjvO_2$ are reflective of changes in CBF only if arterial oxygen saturation and hemoglobin concentration are relatively constant [23].

It has to be recognized that $SjvO_2$ monitors global cerebral oxygenation and may not detect regional ischemia. Another limitation of the technique is the high incidence of artifacts, e.g., because of malpositioning of the catheter tip. Even with a high degree of personal effort, "time of good data quality" is only 40% – 60% [5, 14, 25].

Monitoring of Brain Tissue Oxygen Pressure (PtiO$_2$)

Measurement of brain tissue oxygen pressure in cerebral white matter is a new, promising method for monitoring cerebral oxygenation [10, 14, 27]. $PtiO_2$ can be measured by a Clark-type microcatheter, inserted into the nonlesioned frontal white matter by a specific introducer and fixed on a special skull screw. The catheter is connected to a monitor where the $PtiO_2$ value is given in mm Hg.

Normal values of $PtiO_2$ in the white matter are expected to be in the range of 20 – 40 mm Hg. A $PtiO_2$ below 10 – 15 mm Hg is considered hypoxic, in analogy to the 50 % threshold of jugular venous oxygen saturation [14].

Decreases in $PtiO_2$ can be observed when cerebral perfusion pressure falls below 60 mm Hg, caused by low arterial blood pressure or intracranial hypertension. Forced hyperventilation ($paCO_2$ < 30 mm Hg) may also decrease $PtiO_2$. Insufficient arterial oxygenation (paO_2 < 100 mm Hg) is another reason for a low $PtiO_2$.

$PtiO_2$ monitoring is invasive and not yet introduced into daily clinical routine, but it appears to be a sensitive diagnostic method to follow cerebral oxygenation. In comparison to $SjvO_2$, $PtiO_2$ monitoring is more suitable for long-term measurements because of a low incidence of artifacts. When monitored in nonlesioned brain, a good correlation between global cerebral oxygenation ($SjvO_2$) and regional $PtiO_2$ has been described [14].

The purpose of this study was to compare the three methods available to monitor cerebral oxygenation in patients with severe head injury. The following questions should be answered:

1. Is the method suitable for continuous monitoring of cerebral oxygenation?
2. How sensible is the method in detecting episodes of ischemia and hypoxia, expected to occur with a cerebral perfusion pressure below 60 mm Hg?

Clinical Material and Methods

Patient Population and Management

Seventeen comatose patients with severe head injury were investigated, with an average age of 30 years (range: 14–52 years). On admission, the median Glasgow Coma Scale score was 5 (range: 3–8). All patients had been intubated and ventilated on the scene. After resuscitation, cranial computerized tomography (CCT) was performed. All patients were managed according to a standard protocol:

A PaO_2 greater than 100 mm Hg and a $PaCO_2$ ca. 35 mm Hg was maintained. Intracranial pressure (ICP) was monitored intraparenchymally (Camino Laboratories, San Diego, CA). Medications included fentanyl and midazolam for analogosedation and, if necessary, antibiotic drugs. Hemoglobin concentration was held above 10 g/dl. Intracranial hypertension (ICP > 20 mm Hg) was treated with elevated head positioning, moderate hyperventilation ($PaCO_2$ ca. 30 mm Hg) and mannitol (0.5 g/kg body weight). Efforts were made to hold the cerebral perfusion pressure (CPP) above 70 mm Hg. Barbiturate coma was used only if intracranial hypertension was refractory to the above regimen and it included on-line EEG monitoring.

Multimodal monitoring:

Standard monitoring

The following physiological parameters were continuously monitored for as long as ICP monitoring was required: arterial blood pressure via a radial arterial or femoral artery cannula leveled to the skull base, ICP, cerebral blood pressure (CPP), arterial oxygen saturation (SaO_2), end-tidal CO_2, and body temperature. Measurement of ICP was performed using a fiberoptic intraparenchymal device (Camino Laboratories, San Diego, CA). All parameters were recorded at 1-min intervals.

Cerebral monitoring

$SjvO_2$ *Measurements.* To monitor $SjvO_2$, a No. 5.5 French fiberoptic pulmonary catheter (Opticath, Oximetrix SO_2 Systems, Abbott Laboratories, North Chicago, IL) was inserted into the internal jugular vein through a No. 7.5 French introducer. The tip of the catheter was positioned in the jugular bulb at the C-2 vertebral body, which was verified by X-ray film. The catheter was placed on the right side. The catheter was calibrated in vitro prior to insertion according to the method supplied by the manufacturer. Immediately after insertion, and every 12 h thereafter, in vivo verification of catheter calibration was performed by drawing a blood sample from the catheter and measuring the oxygen saturation on a co-oximeter. If the catheter – and co-oximeter – derived values differed by more than 4%, the catheter was recalibrated and the corresponding data marked as artifacts. To prevent blood clotting, a heparinized saline solution was continuously infused. No medications were given through the catheter.

PtiO$_2$ Measurements. A flexible polarographic Clark-type microcatheter (Licox System, GMS, Kiel, Germany; Paratrend, Wycombe, UK) was inserted into the nonlesioned frontal white matter. The catheter placement was guided by a specific introducer that was tightly fixed on a special skull screw. The insertion depth of the probe was 34 mm (from dura level to the catheter tip). Correct location of the catheter was ascertained by a CCT scan. After removal at the end of monitoring the PtiO$_2$ catheters were checked for drift on room air.

Near-Infrared Spectroscopy. Two NIRS monitors (INVOS 3100, Somanetics and Criticon Cerebral RedOx Research Monitor 2020, Johnson & Johnson, Medical, UK) were tested. INVOS 3100 gives cerebral oxygenation values as regional tissue saturation (rSO$_2$) in percent, the Criticon 2020 as HbO$_2$, Hb, and CytO$_2$ in μmol/l. In 11 patients the "Invos 3100" was used and in six patients the Criticon 2020. In all patients the sensor was fixed tightly on the desinfected dry skin of the right frontal area.

Data Collection

All parameters were stored and analyzed on a multimodal computer system with appropriate software (LabVIEW; National Instruments, Austin, TX), (for a detailed description, see Bardt 1996). All data were reviewed by a physician and artifacts were excluded. The following data were additionally excluded from data analysis:

- SjvO$_2$ values > 75%
- PtiO$_2$ values > 40 mm Hg
- NIRS values > 80%

"Time of good data quality" was calculated by the formula:

- "time of good data quality" [%]=100 – (time of artifacts (min) 100)/total monitoring time (min).

To test the sensitivity of the methods, "critical episodes," defined as a marked decrease in CPP ($<$ 50 mm Hg $\geq$ 5 min) were taken. For correlation analysis the data of 10 patients with continuous PtiO$_2$ and NIRS monitoring and decreases in CPP < 60 mm Hg were taken for following correlations (PtiO$_2$ vs NIRS, CPP vs PtiO$_2$).

Statistical Analysis

Statistical analysis was performed with SigmaStat 3.0 (Jandel Scientific Co-operation, San Rafael, CA). Values are given as the mean ± standard error of mean unless otherwise indicated. A probability value of less than 0.05 was considered significant. Dotted lines appearing in the graphs indicate the 99% prediction interval.

Results

Time Of Monitoring

There were no complications related to the insertion of the $PtiO_2$ and $SjvO_2$ catheter, in particular no bleeding or infection was observed. Continuous data acquisition was possible for $PtiO_2$, $SjvO_2$ and NIRS-INVOS. With the Criticon 2020, cerebral oxygenation could not be measured even after several changes of the sensor position (6 patients). With INVOS 3100 there are data for 10 patients while in one patient no rSO_2 could be monitored.

Duration of monitoring time, before and after artifact exclusion can be taken from Table 1. Mean duration of cerebral oxygenation monitoring was 8.6 days (range: 2.5 to 12 days) for $PtiO_2$, 4.5 days (range: 1.7 to 6 days) for $SjvO_2$ and 4.2 days (0.7 to 5 days) for NIRS-INVOS.

The $PtiO_2$ method had less artifacts compared to the other two methods. Therefore time of good data quality was highest for $PtiO_2$ (95.2%), intermediate for $SjvO_2$ (66.4%), and low for NIRS-INVOS (51.5%).

The most frequent cause for $SjvO_2$-related artifacts was "low light intensity" because of abutment of the catheter tip against the vessel wall, which disappeared when the catheter was flushed. On two occasions catheters were found to be looped in the internal jugular vein and position was corrected by retracting the catheter. In one patient the $PtiO_2$ sensor had to be repositioned and refixed.

Table 1. Cerebral monitoring: duration of measurement before and after artifact exclusion Values of monitoring time are given in days (minutes). "Time of good data" in percent.

	$PtiO_2$ (N=17)	$SjvO_2$ (N=8)	rSO_2 (N=10)
Total monitoring time	84.7 days (121 968 min)	25.5 days (36 720 min)	53.1 days (76 477 min)
Monitoring time after artifact exclusion	80.6 days (116 064 min)	16.9 days (24 336 min)	27.3 days (39 369 min)
"Time of good data"	95.2%	66.4%	51.5%

$PtiO_2$ brain tissue oxygen pressure; $SjvO_2$ oxygen saturation in the jugular venous bulb; rSO_2 regional oxygen saturation (NIRS, INVOS 3100)

Sensitivity of methods to detect decreases in CPP

Twenty-five episodes (820 min) of low CPP were found. In Table 2, the mean values before, at lowest CPP, and after CPP recovery are given. In the majority of cases, a decrease in mean arterial blood pressure was responsible for the low CPP.

The low CPP was followed by a decrease in cerebral oxygenation. This deterioration of cerebral oxygenation, expressed in percentage change ("before versus at the timepoint of minimum cerebral perfusion pressure") was signifi-

Table 2. Parameters of multimodal monitoring of 25 episodes of critically low CPP

	MAP (mm Hg)	ICP (mm Hg)	CPP (mm Hg)	$PtiO_2$ (mm Hg)	$SjvO_2$ (%)	rSO_2 (%)
Before CPP decrease	98.4 ± 7	25.7 ± 8	73.6 ± 4	22.5 ± 8	66.8 ± 7	61.1 ± 3
CPP minimum	72.3 ± 12	31.9 ± 11	41.1 ± 9	14.5 ± 7	63.1 ± 18	59.7 ± 4
CCP recovery	102.8 ± 8.3	22.3 ± 9	81.5 ± 8.3	19.8 ± 8.3	72.2 ± 7.6	62.4 ± 4.6

* Values are given as mean ± standard deviation. MAP, mean arterial pressure; ICP, intracranial pressure; CPP, cerebral perfusion pressure; $PtiO_2$ partial pressure of brain tissue oxygen; $SjvO_2$ jugular venous oxygen saturation; rSO_2 regional tissue oxygen saturation (NIRS)

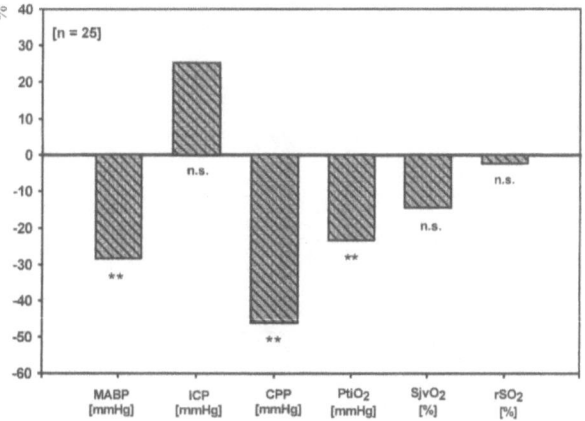

Fig. 1. Multimodal monitoring: changes (in %) of mean arterial pressure (MAP), intracranial pressure (ICP), cerebral perfusion pressure (CPP), partial pressure of brain tissue oxygen ($PtiO_2$), jugular venous saturation ($SjvO_2$), and regional tissue saturation (rSO_2-NIRS) after a decrease in CPP below 50 mm Hg ≥ 5 min

cant for $PtiO_2$, but not for $SjvO_2$ and rSO_2 monitoring (Fig. 1). In individual cases, $SjvO_2$ decreased markedly, while near-infrared spectroscopy revealed only marginal changes in rSO_2 (Fig. 2). $PtiO_2$ monitoring yielded the most consistent data. $PtiO_2$ decreased in all episodes of reduced CPP and even reached hypoxic threshold in 20% of these episodes.

Correlation Analysis

Below a cerebral perfusion pressure threshold of 60 mm Hg, $PtiO_2$ decreases parallel to a decreasing CPP while there was no further improvement of $PtiO_2$ if cerebral perfusion pressure increased above 60 mm Hg (Fig. 3a). This confirms earlier reports by Kiening, who found a significant correlation between CPP and $PtiO_2$ below 60 mm Hg of CPP [14]. No correlation between rSO_2 (NIRS) versus CPP (Fig. 3b) and rSO_2 versus CPP was found.

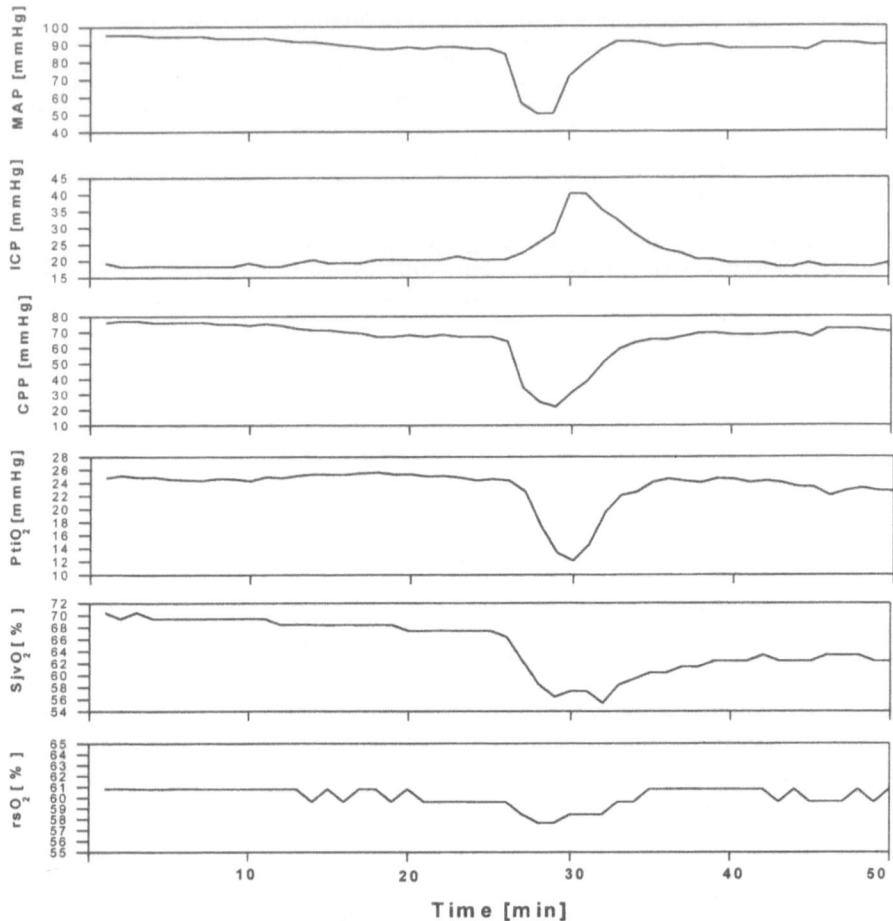

Fig. 2. Multimodal monitoring: effect of cerebral perfusion pressure on cerebral oxygenation ($PtiO_2$, $SjvO_2$, rSO_2-NIRS). This graph shows an individual example. The decrease in cerebral perfusion pressure (caused by a decline in mean arterial blood pressure of 45 mm Hg for 10 minutes) is followed by a subsequent reduction in cerebral oxygenation, expressed as decrease in $PtiO_2$, $SjvO_2$ and rSO_2 (NIRS)

Discussion

It is increasingly being recognized that improved care for severely head-injured patients, directed toward minimizing secondary brain damage is likely to have an impact on reduced mortality and morbidity. Meanwhile, continuous monitoring of mean arterial blood pressure (MABP), ICP, CPP, and arterial pCO_2 (as end-tidal CO_2) is standard monitoring for severely head-injured patients. To detect ischemic and hypoxic episodes, however, additional monitoring of cerebral oxygenation is mandatory. Today, three methods of

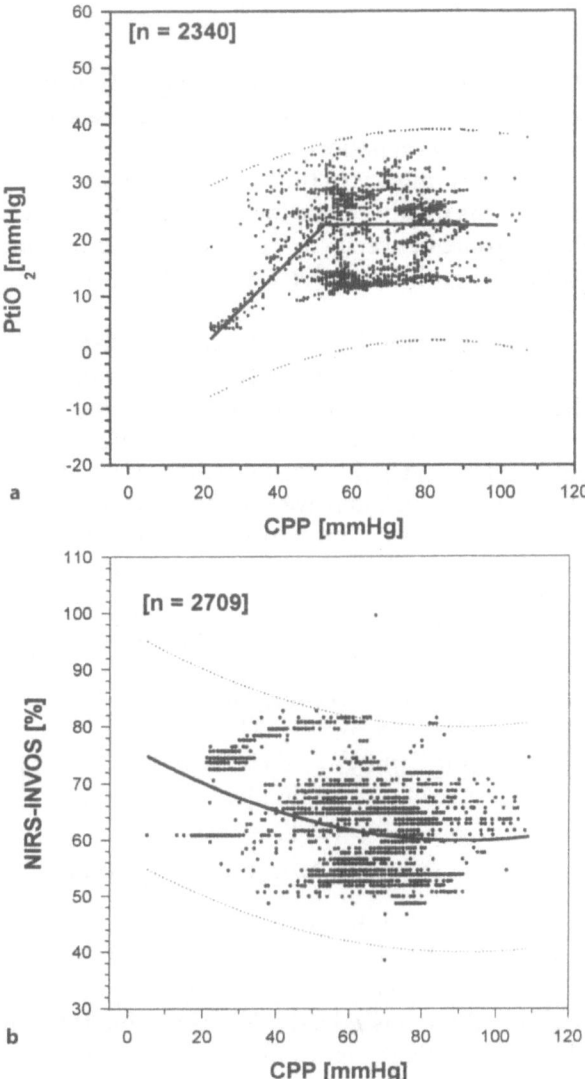

Fig. 3. a Correlation analysis brain tissue oxygen pressure ($PtiO_2$) and cerebral perfusion pressure (CPP). The two lines illustrate the reaction of $PtiO_2$ above and below a critical CPP of 60 mm Hg. **b** Correlation analysis of rSO_2 (NIRS-INVOS) and CPP. No relation is evident

monitoring cerebral oxygenation are available and were tested in patients with severe head injury: monitoring of jugular venous oxygen saturation ($SjvO_2$), monitoring of local brain tissue oxygen pressure ($PtiO_2$) and the near-infrared spectroscopy (NIRS).

Time of Monitoring

The method to monitor cerebral oxygenation most often studied is $SjvO_2$ monitoring. It is generally accepted that this method allows continuous monitoring of cerebral oxygenation [4, 5, 21]. In our study mean $SjvO_2$ monitoring time was 4.5 days which is in the range of other authors [16]. The main point of criticism of this method is the low "time of good data quality". Values known from literature are between 40 – 60% [5, 8, 14]. In this study, "time of good data quality" was slightly better (66.4%) which may be explained by frequent recalibrations.

Another method to follow cerebral oxygenation is near-infrared spectroscopy. The big advantage of NIRS is its noninvasiveness. The majority of studies use NIRS for short-term measurements, e.g., carotid endarterectomy [29]. In patients with severe head injury several technical problems are described, e.g., the long-term fixation of the sensor and the influence of different lighting conditions in the intensive care unit [15]. Also the presence of subgaleal hematomas in the sensor area may disturb measurement since they alter the absorbtion spectrum of the tissue between skin and brain [7, 8].

With the INVOS 3100, the "time of good data quality" was only 51.5%. This is slightly higher than in a comparable study with severely head-injured patients (42.4%; [8]).

Measurement of brain tissue oxygen pressure is the most recently introduced method [13, 14, 27]. The mean duration of $PtiO_2$ monitoring was 8.6 days, varying from 3 to 9 days [14, 27]. "Time of good data quality" was above 90% because of a small number of artifacts.

Sensitivity of Methods to Detect Decreases in CPP

It is well accepted that $SjvO_2$ monitoring is capable of detecting "desaturation episodes" indicating reduced global oxygenation of the brain in patients with severe head injury [4, 5, 21]. Taking all episodes of critically reduced CPP into account, there was a decrease in $SjvO_2$, but it was not significant. This is due to the fact that there were some episodes of low CPP that were not reflected by $SjvO_2$ decreases.

It could be that the CPP decrease was not sufficient to affect global cerebral oxygenation. By analyzing such individual episodes of CPP decrease, it appears that the intensity of CPP reduction is more important than the duration of a low CPP.

In NIRS, there was a wide variance of the baseline values (rSO_2 between 49% – 81%). The normal range is supposed to be between 59% and 79% [3, 23]. The mean decrease in cerebral oxygenation during episodes of critical reduction in CPP measured by NIRS was marginal 1.9 (−5 to 0)% only. This is similar to the rSO_2 decrease of 2 (7 to −9)% during clipping in carotid endarterectomy. In addition, there was no relation between rSO_2 and cerebral perfusion pressure.

The sensitivity of $PtiO_2$ monitoring in relation to decreases in CPP has already been studied: Parallel to a reduction of CPP, cerebral oxygenation deteriorated measured with $PtiO_2$ and $SjvO_2$ [14]. In this study, $PtiO_2$ decreased in all episodes of reduced CPP. In ca. 20% it even reached the hypoxic threshold (< 10 mm Hg).

Conclusion

Continuous monitoring of cerebral oxygenation can be achieved by monitoring of jugular venous oxygen saturation ($SjvO_2$) and by measurement of brain tissue oxygen pressure ($PtiO_2$) but not with near infrared spectroscopy (NIRS).

$PtiO_2$ and $SjvO_2$ monitoring detects episodes of ischemia and hypoxia caused by a decrease in cerebral perfusion pressure. When CPP is restored, cerebral oxygenation improves. A reduction of cerebral perfusion pressure (below 50 mm Hg > 5 min) is reflected by a deterioration of cerebral oxygenation.

NIRS techniques available have numerous technical problems and can momentarily not be used to detect decreases in CPP. Thus, the routine use of near-infrared spectroscopy to monitor cerebral oxygenation in patients with severe head injury cannot be currently recommended.

References

1. Bardt TF, Unterberg AW, Kiening KL, Schneider GH, Lanksch WR (1997) Multimodal cerebral monitoring in comatose head-injured patients. J Clin Monit (submitted)
2. Chan KH, Dearden NM, Miller JD (1993) Multimodality monitoring as a guide to treatment of intracranial hypertension after severe head injury. Neurosurgery 32: 547–553
3. Colier WNJM, van Haaren NJCW, Oeseburg B (1995) A comparative study of two near infrared spectrophotometers for the assessment of cerebral haemodynamics. Acta Anaesthesiol Scand 39 [Suppl 107]: 101–105
4. Cruz J (1988) Continuous versus serial global cerebral haemometabolic monitoring: application in acute brain trauma. Acta Neurochir Suppl (Wien) 42: 35–39
5. Dearden NM (1991) Jugular bulb venous oxygen saturation in the management of severe head injury. Curr Opin Anaesth 4: 279–286
6. Dearden NM, Midgley S (1993) Technical considerations in continuous jugular venous oxygenation saturation measurements. In: Unterberg AW, Schneider GH, Lanksch WR (eds) Monitoring of cerebral blood flow and metabolism in intensive care. Acta Neurochir Suppl (Wien) 59: 91–97
7. Firbank M, Arridge SR, Schweiger M, Delpy DT (1996) An investigation of light transport through scattering bodies with non-scattering regions. Phys Med Biol 41: 767–783
8. Gopinath SP, Robertson CS, Contant CF, Narayan RK, Grossman RG, Chance BSO (1995) Early detection of delayed traumatic intracranial hematomas using near-infrared spectroscopy. J Neurosurg 83 (3): 438
9. Graham DI, Ford I, Adams JH, Doyle D, Teasdale GM, Lawrence AE, Mc Lellan DR (1989) Ischaemic brain damage is still common in fatal non-missile head injury. J Neurol Neurosurg Psychiatry 52: 346–350
10. Hoffmann WE, Charbel FT, Edelmann G (1996) Brain tissue oxygen, carbon dioxide and pH in neurosurgical patients at risk for ischemia. Anesth Anal 82: 582–586
11. Jøbsis FF (1977) Noninvasive, infrared monitoring of cerebral and myocardial oxygen sufficiency and circulatory parameters. Science 198: 1264–1267

12. Jones MD, Traystman RJ, Simmons MA, Molteni RA: Effects of changes in arterial O_2 content on cerebral blood flow in the lamb. Am J Physiol (2): H209–H215
13. Kiening KL, Härtl R, Unterberg AW, Schneider GH, Bardt TF, Lanksch RW (1997) Brain tissue PO_2-monitoring in comatose patients: implications for therapy. Neurol Res (in press)
14. Kiening KL, Unterberg AW, Bardt TF, Schneider GH, Lanksch RW (1996) Monitoring of cerebral oxygenation in severely head-injured patients: brain tissue PO_2 vs jugular venous oxygen saturation. J Neurosurg 1996; 85: 751–757
15. Kirkpatrick PJ, Smielewski P, Czosnyka M, Menon DK, Pickard JD (1995) Near-infrared spectroscopy use in patients with head injury. J Neurosurg 83: 963–970
16. Lewis SB, Myburgh JA, Thornton EL, Reilly PL (1996) Cerebral oxygenation monitoring by near-infrared spectroscopy is not clinically useful in patients with severe closed-head injury: A comparison with jugular venous bulb oximetry. Crit Care Med 24 (8): 1334–1338
17. Litscher G, Schwarz G, Jobstmann R, Klein G, Neumann J, Prietl B (1995) Nichtinvasive Überwachung der regionalen zerebralen Sauerstoffsättigung – Erfahrungen aus der Intensivmedizin. Biomed Technik 40: 70–75
18. Maas AIR, Fleckenstein W, De Jong DA, van Santbrink H (1993) Monitoring cerebral oxygenation: experimental studies and preliminary clinical results of continuous monitoring of cerebrospinal fluid and brain tissue oxygen tension. In: Unterberg AW, Schneider GH, Lanksch WR (eds) Monitoring of cerebral blood flow and metabolism in intensive care. Acta Neurochir Suppl (Wien) 59: 50–57
19. Obrist WD, Marion DW (1996) Xenon techniques for CBF measurement in clinical head injury. In: Narayan RK, Wilberger JE, Povlishock JT (eds) Neurotrauma. McGraw-Hill, 33: 471–485
20. Overgaard J, Mosdal C, Tweed WA (1981) Cerebral circulation after head injury. Part 3: Does reduced regional cerebral blood flow determine recovery of brain function after blunt head injury? J Neurosurg 55: 63–74
21. Robertson CS (1993) Desaturation episodes after severe head injury: influence on outcome. Acta Neurochir Suppl 59: 98–101
22. Robertson CS (1993) Nitrous oxide saturation technique for CBF measurement. In: Narayan, Wilberger, Povlishock (eds) Neurotrauma. McGraw-Hill 34: 487–501
23. Robertson CS, Narayan RK, Gokaslan ZL, Pahwan R, Grossman RG, Caram P, Allen E (1989) Cerebral arteriovenous oxygen difference as an estimate of cerebral blood flow in comatose patients. J Neurosurg 70: 222–230
24. Schneider GH, v. Helden A, Lanksch WR, Unterberg A (1995) Continuous monitoring of jugular bulb oxygen saturation in comatose patients – therapeutic implications. Acta Neurochir (Wien) 134: 71–75
25. Schwarz G, Litscher G, Kleinert R, Jobstmann R (1996) Cerebral oxymetry in dead subjects. J Neurosurg Anesth 8 (3): 189–193
26. Sheinberg M, Kanter MJ, Robertson CS, Contant CF, Narayan RK, Grossman RG (1992) Continuous monitoring of jugular venous oxygen saturation in head-injured patients. J Neurosurg 76: 212–217
27. Van Santbrink H, Maas AIR, Avezaat CJJ (1996) Continuous monitoring of partial pressure of brain tissue oxygen in patients with severe head injury. Neurosurgery 38: 21–32
28. Wahr JA, Tremper, KK (1995) Noninvasive oxygen monitoring techniques. Crit-Care-Clin. Jan; 11 (1): 199–217
29. Williams IM, Picton A, Farrell A, Mead GE, Mortimer AJ, McCollum CN (1994) Light-reflective cerebral oxymetry and jugular bulb venous oxygen saturation during carotid endarterectomy. Brit J Surg 81: 1291–1295
30. Woodman T, Robertson CS (1996) Jugular venous oxygen saturation monitoring. In: Narayan RK, Wilberger JE, Povlishock JT (eds) Neurotrauma. McGraw-Hill 36: 521

14 Traumatic Lesions of Cranial Nerves in Head-Injured Patients

M. Samii and C. Matthies

Introduction

The acute management of head injuries is dominated by the impending danger of brain compression and herniation, cerebral edema, and compromise of vital vegetative functions. Attention is directed only secondarily to focal circumscribed lesions of the cranial nerves. Fortunately, these are rare; still, it is important to diagnose them early in order to take the adequate steps of treatment. Among all the cranial nerves possibly involved in head trauma, the early detection, exact timing of exploration, and treatment are of utmost importance for the optic, facial, and cochlear nerves.

Blindness from head injury is a catastrophic lesion that can be prevented in specific cases successfully, however, only by early detection and management within the first hours. Facial nerve paralysis is the most frequent and one of the most devastating peripheral nerve injuries. The functional compromise leads to dropping of the eye brow and disturbed vision, to frequent painful inflammations due to malfunction of the lacrimal gland, to lagophthalmos, and sometimes to keratitis with scarring and secondary blurred vision. The loss of movement and of control of the involved mouth angle causes impaired speech and expression. Still, most patients suffer at first from the loss of their individual "mirror image" and judge the cosmetic disturbance as unbearable. Bilateral deafness may occur as a result of bilateral temporal bone fractures. Deafness can be masked for long during the management of head-injured patients with disturbed consciousness.

Historical Aspects of Nerve Surgery and Reconstruction. Since the successful grafting of peripheral nerves in man in the last century the fate of patients with nerve lesions has changed remarkably. Although a restitutio ad integrum cannot be achieved, a satisfying outcome may be obtained for some sensory and motor nerves. Around 1900 the attempts for restoration of facial nerve function were intensified. In 1927 Bunnell's pioneer work [6] of intratemporal facial nerve surgery was a breakthrough demonstrating that readaptation of facial nerve ends intratemporally is possible, and that, moreover, free nerve grafts lead to reinnervation of the facial nerve within its temporal course. Cardwell in 1938 [7] and Maxwell [42, 43] and Conley [9–11] in the 1950s worked on the extracranial reconstruction of the facial nerve in trauma and in parotid gland tumors. Conley started using the greater auricular nerve as a free graft and put a cylinder around the site of nerve adaptation. Especially since Dott's [19] invention of an intracranial-extracranial nerve transplantation, which proved that nerve reconstruction intradurally just distally to the ganglion/nucleus is feasible. This led to further developments such as the intracranial [52–54, 58] and intracranial-intratemporal [20] nerve reconstruction as well as that of other cranial nerves, namely the trigeminal [26, 51, 57] and the oculomotoric nerves [16, 23, 40, 60). Modern microsurgical techniques, refined during the past three decades, have greatly enhanced this development.

Long-Term Patient Guidance and Management. The treatment options at hand for the patient with cranial nerve lesions are sufficient and in general successful [30, 48, 55, 60, 65] to prevent long-term serious disabilities or devastating cosmetic disturbances. However, the patient must endure a difficult waiting period until the first signs of nerve recovery appear up. The functional deficits and cosmetic disturbances as well as the (latent) anxieties about possible failure of reinnervation might for some time produce a state of depression. During this period the continuous availability of a specialist and regular control examinations are necessary. Only in this way can the patient and the relatives be assured that the course is within the normal range, and that the steps of controls and treatment will lead to a satisfying result. The providing of such information to family physicians and cooperating disciplines should be a basic principle and is of tremendous help.

Principles and Discussion of Nerve Reconstructive Techniques. An advanced neurosurgeon with thorough personal experience in nerve surgery should participate in each nerve reconstructive procedure. Only in this way can the lack of knowledge in these statistically rare interventions be overcome. Substantial experience is necessary in general grafting techniques and in the anatomy and texture of the cranial nerves. The most proximal part of the facial nerve at the brainstem consists mainly of nerve fibers with only little surrounding connective sheath, making it extremely vulnerable and difficult to handle. Most important is the identification and preparation of vital proximal and distal nerve stumps. It is not easy to judge the viability of a nerve stump, and this difficulty may be the major reason for reports of failures in grafting within the cerebellopontine angle (CPA) [30, 32, 65]. In some cases the diagnosis of a complete loss of a proximal nerve stump requires a reanimation procedure and prevents an unsuccessful grafting.

Furthermore, it is similarly difficult to perform the nerve adaptation within the CPA at the pulsating brainstem. The nerve stumps need to be inspected and prepared carefully. They must be free of any degenerated segments and show vital axons trimmed to similar lengths, and they should not be distorted against each other. On adaptation of the nerve stumps any distorsion against one another, overlapping of axons, and tension [51, 57] are avoided. A longer transplant is to be taken instead of an adaptation with tension. Experience shows that transplant length of 0.5 or 15 cm leads to good results. Stephanian et al. [65] found no affect of transplant length on the final outcome. Fixation of the adapted nerve stumps is performed by fine sutures without tearing or distorting the fibers. For an increase in stability, a little fibrin glue may be applied outside on the adaptation site, but no glue should drop between the axon endings. This entire process must prevent any further trauma to the nerves. Tearing, rotation, and many sutures are all factors enhancing the process of scarring and are therefore to be avoided. In especially delicate cases with difficulty of broad access to the site of transplantation, the whole adaptation may be performed with external fibrin glue instead of suturing; this leads to the same quality of results when performed correctly [55].

Regarding the nerve graft, the selection of the sural nerve instead of the frequently chosen greater auricular nerve offers the advantage of not impairing the sensory function at the craniocervical region, as the sural sensory deficit at the foot is generally better accepted.

The management of each cranial nerve is briefly summarized below with special emphasis on those that are amenable to reconstruction and those with the most frequent indications for microsurgical interventions.

Olfactory Nerve

The olfactory nerve is endangered in frontobasal traumas with fractures involving the cribriform plate, and secondarily in surgical treatment of these lesions.

Diagnosis is made clinically on thorough neurological testing of smelling of aromatic substances (vanillin, coffee). In general this is feasible only after the acute trauma phase, and after the patient's consciousness has become adequate. An objective assessment may then be supported by olfactory evoked potentials [41].

The indication for surgery is not led by anosmia or olfactory dys- or malfunction but only by the necessity to treat persistent cerebrospinal fluid leakage. Evaluation by endonasal endoscopy [8] can be helpful without further endangering the olfactory nerve. No reconstruction of the olfactory system is possible. The decompression from bone fragments or hematoma may support the recovery of a lesioned nerve in continuity.

In most cases the repair of a dural leak may be accomplished by the rhinosurgical approach by the otorhinolaryngological team, with the advantage of not touching the olfactory nerve. If in extensive destruction of bone and dura a subfrontal exposure of the anterior skull base is indicated, special care is to be taken to preserve any parts of the olfactory fila, bulb, and tractus and their vascularization [21].

Optic Nerve

The optic nerve is endangered in frontobasal traumas with fractures involving the orbit, especially the orbital base, the paranasal sinuses, namely the maxillary and ethmoidal sinuses. In addition, direct or indirect trauma to the eyeball and orbital cavity, such as acceleration-translation trauma due to a hit by a fast vehicle or a fall must be considered.

Diagnosis is made clinically and radiologically. Mono- or binocular hematoma arouses suspicion. Inspection of the eyeball and the pupil are sometimes impossible due to the progressing extreme local swelling. This inspection is indicated as early as possible on admittance to the emergency unit. In order to differentiate the causes of mydriasis – either oculomotor nerve compression due to cerebral herniation at the tentorial notch or direct optic nerve trauma – direct and indirect reactions to light are tested. If the dilated pupil is nonreactive to direct light but shows some indirect contraction on light to the other eye, a direct optic nerve trauma is most likely. A thorough emergency neuro-ophthalmological examination with evaluation of the vitrous body, fundus, intrabulbar pressure, and optical axis are indicated. The optic nerve can be identified by computed tomography (CT) in most cases. A coarse discontinuity is detected as well as a compressive lesion such as retrobulbar or optic sheath hematoma. At bone window CT the fractured parts of the orbital cavity, any dislocation of fragments, and especially a destroyed orbital base are analyzed as well as the patency of the optic canal. If all these diagnostic measures fail to clarify the state of the optic nerve, visual evoked potentials (VEPs) to flash stimulation appear to provide reliable information on function within the visual pathway [14].

The indication for surgery is given at urgent suspicion of an optic nerve compression within the first 6 – 12 h, although the outcome is a matter of discussion [12, 46].

In medial lesions, in most instances a transethmoidal approach, is sufficient to perform a decompression of the optic nerve. Depending on the extension of the space-occupying lesion, especially for the optic sheath or in large retrobulbar lesions, a frontolateral exposure for decompression of the optic nerve by microsurgical technique is the most effective way. In cases of multiple foreign bodies penetrating into the orbit, computer-assisted surgery may facilitate their identification and removal [35]. Reconstruction and repositioning of the orbit and adjusting paranasal sinuses is rarely necessary in the acute phase but is to be planned along with otorhinolaryngologists and maxillofacial surgeons.

Despite a successful nerve decompression or in only partial slight optic nerve lesion secondary visual disturbance may be caused later after the trauma due to chronic open angle glaucoma [66] or posttraumatic lens opacification [4].

Oculomotor, Trochlear, and Abducens Nerves

The oculomotoric nerves are endangered mainly in involvement of the cavernous sinus, by carotid cavernous fistulas or secondary inflammatory thrombosis. In both situations the symptoms of oculomotoric paresis occur at some delay after the trauma or are even difficult to relate to a previous trauma. In rare cases mesencephalic hemorrhage [24] or hemorrhage at the midbrain exit site [2] of the oculomotor nerve may produce partial or complete oculomotor palsy.

Diagnosis of carotid cavernous fistula is made clinically on inspection of the swollen, pulsating eye, exophthalmus, conjunctival injection, fundoscopy with swollen or pulsating retinal veins and on auscultation of the skull and eye with a pulse synchronous murmur. Conventional and/or magnetic resonance imaging (MRI) angiography confirms the diagnosis. Treatment by open surgery or by interventional endovascular occlusion of the carotid cavernous fistula is indicated only in some cases that do not subside spontaneously. During this waiting period regular ophthalmological control is indispensible because loss of vision is one of the major dangers. Recovery of nerve functions usually follows the closure of the fistula.

Diagnosis of inflammatory thrombosis of the cavernous sinus is evident by the painful ophthalmoplegia, swollen eye lids, papillary edema, combination of neurological deficits, severe general disease (possibly increased intracranial pressure) and MRI findings. Treatment is only conservative, by high-dose specific antibiotics.

Diagnosis of traumatic tear or hemorrhage in the nuclear or nerve exit region of the mesencephalon is extremely rare and can be displayed sometimes by MRI.

Surgery will be indicated in a minority of cases. Most experiences with reconstruction of these nerves have so far been gained from surgery of extensive skull base tumors [16, 23, 40, 60]. Whether reconstruction is feasible and the chances of recovery are comparable, if traction trauma has severed the nerve segments, is to be awaited.

Trigeminal Nerve

The nerve is endangered in skull base traumas and in direct face traumas. Temporal bone fractures radiating to the foramina of the sphenoid bone, at the floor of the middle fossa, may lead to tearing or interruption of the trigeminal nerve branches. Direct soft tissue lesions of the face, complex dislocating orbital fractures, maxillary or mandibular fractures can also cause trigeminal nerve lesions.

Diagnosis is based on clinical exploration of any decrease, loss or dysfunction of each trigeminal branch and on radiological diagnosis. Early evaluation and follow-up may be performed additionally – on an objective basis – by quantitative thermography of the sensory and sympathetic function [50].

Priority indication for surgery is given to the repair of the ophthalmic nerve to prevent keratitis neuroparalytica with subsequent ulcerations, scarring, and functional blindness [51, 57]. A retroganglionic damage of the ophthalmic branch can be treated by combination with a cutaneous nerve such as the major occipital nerve. At first, the major occipital nerve is exposed; then the orbital roof is opened via a frontolateral epidural approach, and the ophthalmic nerve can be exposed and proximally transsected after incision of the periorbital capsule. A sural graft is connected to the distal stump of the ophthalmic nerve and then led outside the skull to be connected with the proximal segment of the occipital nerve. Recovery of sensation may be awaited after about 6 months.

Indication for reconstruction of the inferior alveolar nerve is given if the anesthesia of the lower lip leads to difficulty on coordination or recurrent trauma by chewing. Surgery is performed as a joint performance of neurosurgeons and maxillofacial surgeons. At first the proximal and distal nerve ends at the mandibular and mental foramina are identified and marked; the bony reconstruction is the carried out, followed by nerve reconstruction with a nerve graft [13, 26, 51, 57].

Facial Nerve

Causes of facial nerve paralysis in severe head trauma include intrapontine hemorrhage, secondary pontine hypoxia, avulsion from the brainstem, interruption or squeezing of the nerve along its anatomical course from bone fragments by temporal bone fractures [28], extracranial sharp or blunt traumas [63], traumatic pseudoaneurysm of the superficial temporal artery [39], and additional retrograde degeneration. The incidence of traumatic facial nerve lesions among other causes for facial nerve reconstruction ranges from 10 % [55] to 18 % [17].

Diagnosis is made clinically on inspection of the face on rest and on movement and on inquiring about vegetative activity such as lacrimal and nasal gland functions. Electromyography is indicated repeatedly over 6 months to recognize first signs of spontaneous reinnervation.

Indication for surgery is given in case of known nerve discontinuity or of destruction of the facial nucleus; otherwise it is to be scheduled in case of persistence of paralysis after 6 to a maximum of 12 months. The waiting period should be reduced in case of fast progressing muscular atrophy.

Depending on the clinical and radiological diagnosis of the site of the facial nerve lesion, intracranial, intratemporal or extracranial exposure and reconstruction of the facial nerve or facial nerve reanimation with a donor nerve are indicated.

Nuclear Facial Nerve Lesions

Nuclear facial nerve lesions are due to traumatic concussion with hemorrhage, edema, and/or hypoxia of the facial nucleus within the pons. In the acute phase of such brainstem lesions, antiedematous treatment, optimal oxygenation, and microcirculation need to be provided. In this most proximal type of a peripheral facial lesion a waiting period for possible recovery is scheduled for 6 months; physiotherapy is applied, and electromyographic controls are carried out at 1- to 2-month intervals. After persistence, depending on the speed of progression of the muscular atrophy, a reanimation procedure is indicated. If there are additional serious caudal cranial nerve lesions, a facio-facial combination is recommended. Otherwise, in the majority of cases the hypoglossal-facial combination is the method of choice [36].

Facio-facial nerve combination (as described in [59, 71]) is used in patients in whom no other cranial nerve shall or can be sacrified, such as in caudal cranial nerve palsy. The procedure is based on the knowledge that one-third to one-half of the plexiform facial nerve branches on the healthy side of the face may be cut without discernible deficit. These branches are connected via nerve transplants to the corresponding branches of the plegic side. As the innervation pattern shows a great interindividual variance, intraoperative electrophysiological identification of the branches and their functions may be helpful. We choose the zygomatic branches, the strongest among the facial branches, related to both the orbicularis oculi and the orbicularis oris muscles, and expose them by 2-cm-long incisions. The reinnervation must be anticipated to take rather long, sometimes more than 1 year, and to be rather weak. Therefore additional plastic surgery, such as Pitanguy's oval skin resection at the nasolabial fold, temporalis, or masseter muscle transfer are may be performed along with the nerve combination [5, 47].

Hypoglossal-facial combination (as invented by Koerte in 1903 [36]) is performed by combining the proximal part of the hypoglossal nerve (gained below the digastric muscle) with the distal segment of the facial nerve at the stylomastoid process. Microscopic nerve adaptation is performed and stabilized by two 10/0 sutures. In addition to the conventional physiotherapy, the patient is guided to exercise all movements with special tongue movements in various directions towards the gums. Within 1–2 years facial movements become independent from voluntary tongue movements. To minimize the side affects of hypoglossal palsy after hypoglossal-facial combination, some authors [1, 15] have performed combinations with only a part of the hypoglossal nerve or combined the distal part of the hypoglossal nerve with the ansa cervicalis. In our experience, only a mild hypotrophy of the tongue occurs, and speech and food intake are impaired for the first days but are compensated very fast.

Differential Indication of Reanimation Procedures. Donor nerves used for reanimation procedures are the accessory, hypoglossal, and contralateral facial nerves. While the accessory-facial-nerve anastomosis gives evident reinnervation of the facial muscles, the functional and cosmetic results are poor because the innervation is sufficient only on movement of the shoulder. The gross shoulder movements tend not to equal the fine and differentiated pattern of facial innervation. Hypoglossal-facial reanimation entails the chance of strong reliable reinnervation. 74% of patients achieve reinnervation of House-Brackmann grade III [29]; moreover, the results would all be this good in all patients if they were referred early enough, i. e., within 1 year after the onset of palsy. Probably the close connection between the hypoglossal and the facial cortical representation is the reason for the good reinnervation patterns. Kunihiro [38] reported serviceable reinnervation in 25 of 27 treated patients (93%); the results were postulated to be better in cases of early treatment within 3 months than those treated after 12 months.

Far Proximal Lesions Proximal to the Ganglion Geniculi/at the CPA

In complete facial nerve paralysis with loss of lacrimal function the lesion of the facial nerve is most likely proximal to the ganglion geniculi, i. e., it is either intratemporal, at the level of the internal auditory canal, or within the CPA.

In the acute phase medical treatment is useful according to a scheme to treat (a) the neural edema and (b) the disturbed microcirculation. Dexamethasone, hydroxy-ethyl-starch infusion and vasoactive substances such as nimodipine or pentoxifyllin are administered for 10 days intravenously. Neurosurgical treatment is mostly not required in this period. If there is a temporal fracture, cerebrospinal fluid leakage, mastoid fluid retention and middle ear effusion may result. These need at first prevention of infection by antibiotics and then, if leakage does not stop by itself, a plasty with fascia or periosteum within the first weeks after trauma.

In the waiting phase physiotherapy and regular electromyography are performed. If facial paralysis persists over 6 – 10 months with progressing muscular atrophy, the ongoing degeneration necessitates nerve exploration and reconstruction.

Surgical Exploration at the Cerebellopontine Angle. In far proximal lesions pure intratemporal nerve exposure is not sufficient to obtain vital nerve stumps for reconstruction, but nerve exposure at the CPA is indicated. In the supine position with the head mildly anteflected and rotated to the contralateral side or in the semisitting position with the head anteflected and rotated by 30° to the involved side, a lateral suboccipital craniotomy is performed within the angle formed by the transverse and the sigmoid sinuses. After dura opening in a lateral convex shape, first the cerebellomedullary cistern is opened for draining of cerebrospinal fluid, and then the cerebellum can be mildly retracted medially. On inspection of the course of the facial nerve from the brainstem to the entrance at the internal auditory canal the following observations may be made.

Loss of the Proximal Nerve Segment. Either the most proximal part of the nerve is avulsed, or the most proximal part of the nerve is present but completely degenerated due to retrograde degeneration after further distal tearing. In these circumstances no proximal nerve stump is available for reconstruction via transplantation, but a nerve reanimation is indicated, as described above by the hypoglossal-facial combination or facio-facial combination.

A typical case of a temporal facial nerve lesion in a temporal bone fracture with retrograde nerve degeneration is presented by Fig. 1, where hypoglossal-facial combination was performed.

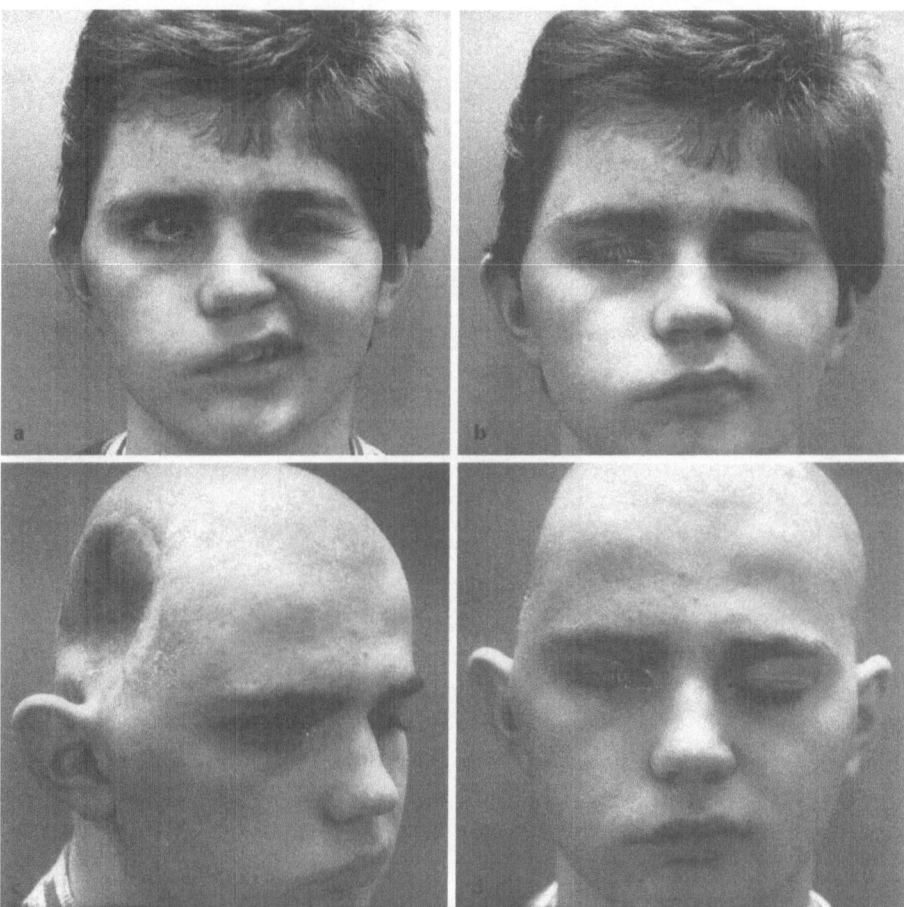

Fig. 1a–h. This 17-year-old patient sustained a severe head injury and needed emergency evacuation of an intracranial hematoma and osteoclastic decompression. **a, b** A right temporal bone fracture caused deafness and facial paralysis. **c, d** At referral to our unit 11 months later three operations were performed: (**a**) facial nerve exploration at the cerebellopontine

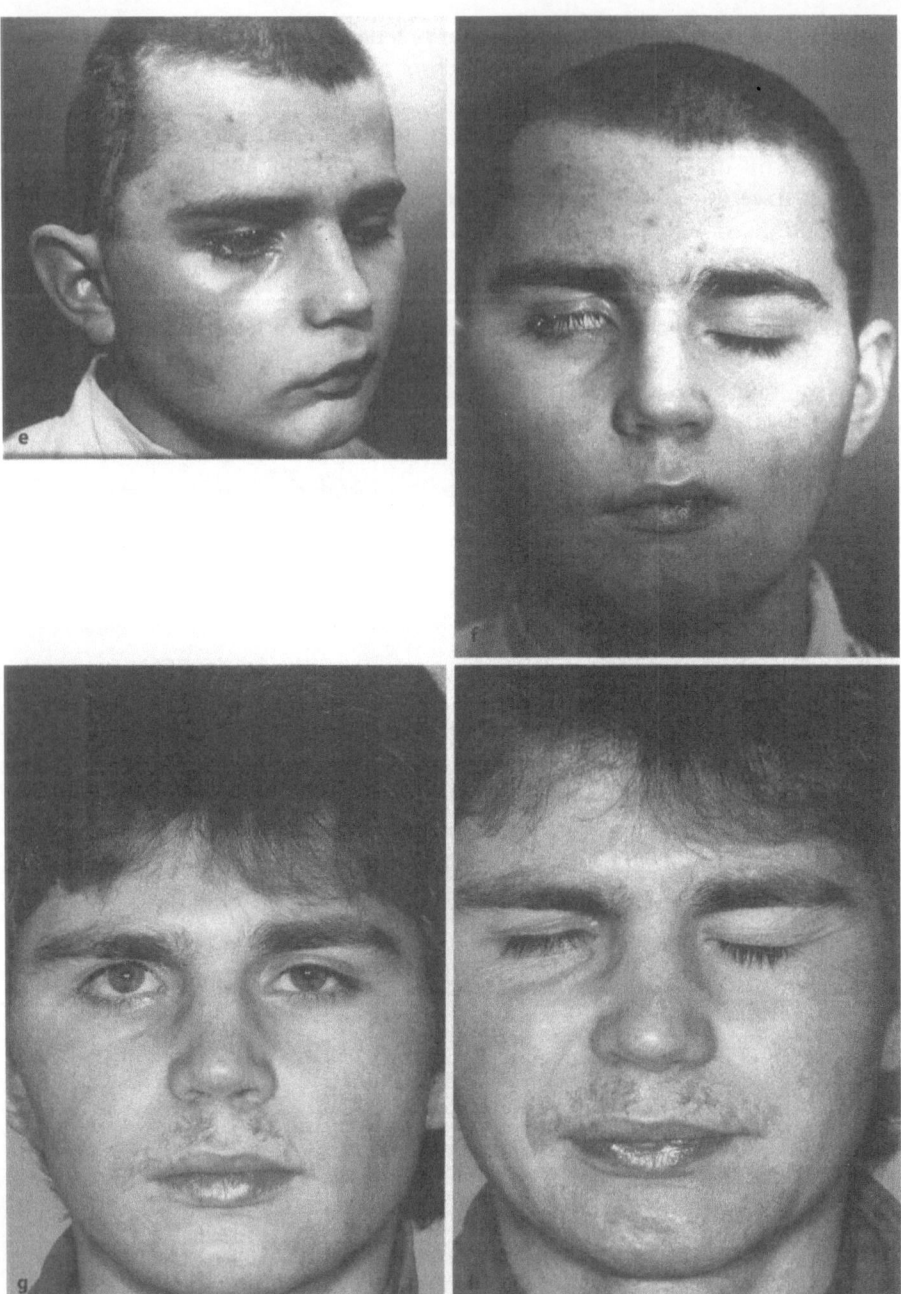

angle revealed retrograde nerve degeneration and no adequate stump at the brainstem; (**b**) a hypoglossal-facial combination was carried out; (**c**) the frontotemporal defect was reconstructed with a methyl-methacrylate plasty (**e, f**). **g, h** Satisfactory facial reinnervation within 2 years is documented with good symmetry on rest and on movement, with complete eye closure and mouth angle control

Interruption of the Facial Nerve Within the CPA. The most proximal part of the nerve is present, but a degeneration or interruption is visible medial to the porus of the internal auditory canal (IAC). The internal auditory canal usually needs to be opened by drilling off the posterior wall, until a healthy nerve segment is exposed. The degenerated parts must be removed, and the gap is bridged by a nerve transplant of 1–3 cm for an intracranial nerve reconstruction within the CPA

Interruption of the Facial Nerve Within the CPA and Temporal Segment. The most proximal part of the facial nerve is present, and some degeneration or interruption is found towards the IAC. Even after opening of the IAC no vital nerve segment is identified. Mastoidotomy or mastoidectomy is then performed to expose the intratemporal nerve segment. A nerve transplant of 5- to 8-cm is prepared, and an intracranial-intratemporal reconstruction is carried out. In rare cases the whole intratemporal segment is found to be degenerated. If there is a history of recurrent mastoiditis or middle ear infections, on the other hand, it may be wise to leave the temporal bone untouched and rather expose the facial nerve at its extracranial segment at the stylomastoid foramen. Then an intracranial-extracranial reconstruction by 12- to 15-cm transplant is performed according to Dott [19].

Intratemporal Lesion Distal to the Ganglion Geniculi. In complete facial nerve paralysis with persistent lacrimal function the lesion of the facial nerve is most likely distal to the ganglion geniculi. The greater petrosal nerve activating, via the pterygoid-palatinal ganglion – the lacrimal and nasal glands – is still intact. The most frequent cause, a temporal fracture, rarely gives rise to a persistent cerebrospinal fluid leak and therefore rarely needs neurosurgical intervention.

In the acute phase medical treatment is useful according to the scheme described above. In the waiting phase physiotherapy and electromyography controls must be guaranteed. After persistence of paralysis over 6–10 months exploration and reconstruction are indicated.

In surgical exploration and nerve reconstruction of the temporal segment the patient is placed in the supine position with the head slightly anteflected and rotated to the contralateral side, and a partial mastoidectomy is perfomed to expose the facial nerve in its temporal course. If an interruption or a neuromatous thickening is found, this part is excised. As soon as a viable proximal and distal nerve stump have been prepared, the gap can be bridged by a free nerve graft, thereby forming an intratemporal nerve reconstruction. If the whole distal segment is destroyed by thickening and scarring, the facial nerve is prepared at its exit at the stylomastoid foramen. An intratemporal-extracranial reconstruction is then performed.

Extracranial Facial Nerve Lesions in the Face and Ear Regions

In the acute phase, in obviously circumscribed lesions generally due to sharp knife or glass trauma, acute treatment is required for hemostasis, prevention of infections, and enabling favorable wound healing in this delicate area. As general surgeons are faced with these lesions in the majority of cases, they should know that – apart from cleaning the wound from any foreign bodies and perfect closure – they should not interfere by searching for any visible nerve fibers or even try "to mark the nerve with clips." All these procedures would rather add further trauma to the nerve and might reduce the vital parts of the nerve further. In short, any such maneuvers render subsequent neurosurgical interventions more difficult and possibly less advantageous.

Moreover, it is not sensible to perform an early nerve exploration and readaptation of interrupted nerve segments. Even if at early surgery we find nerve discontinuity, the viability of the nerve stumps is extremely difficult and unreliable to be judged at that phase. The trauma leads to edematous changes, and in general a larger part of the nerve degenerates during the next weeks if it is handled in this critical period. The likelihood of spontaneous nerve recovery is rather increased if the nerve is merely decompressed from foreign bodies or a hematoma and protected from any further "trauma" such as moving and stretching.

After a waiting period with regular physiotherapy and electromyography controls, palsies after blunt trauma usually recover spontaneously. A seemingly sharp penetrating infra-auricular lesion revealed to be more of a blunt

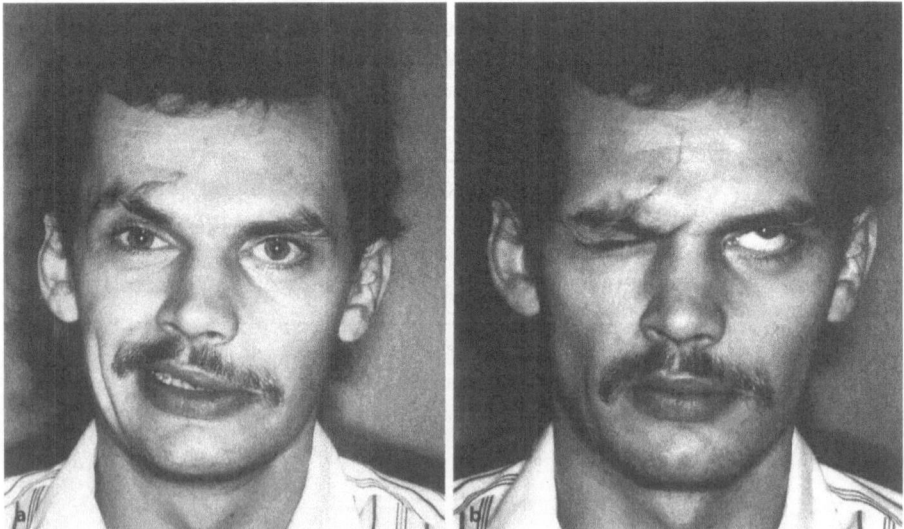

Fig. 2. After a head injury with concussion and two stab wounds at the right front above the eye (**a**) and at the left ear (**d**) this young man presented with a facial palsy (**b, c**). The wounds had been cleared from several pieces of glass of a beer bottle and had healed well (**a, d**).

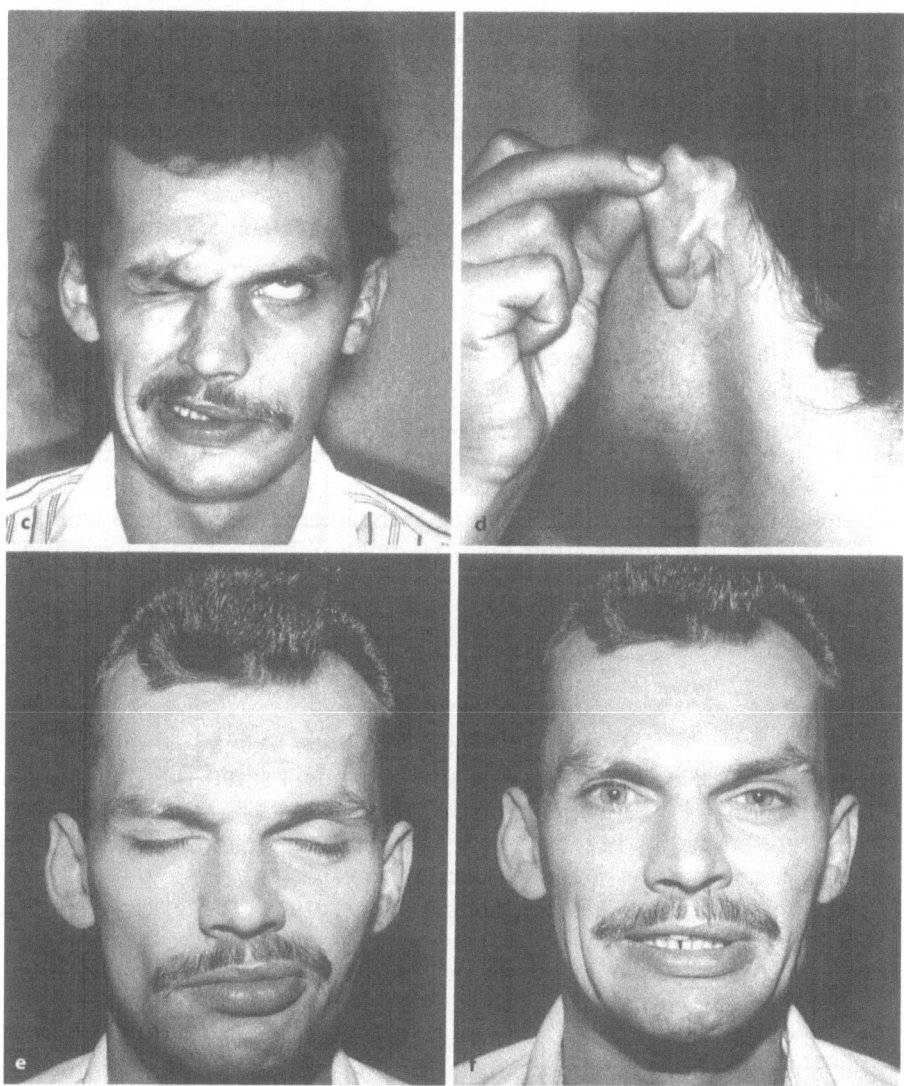

Although there was no knowledge about the exact depth of the infra-auricular penetrating trauma and potential facial nerve discontinuity, awaiting spontaneous recovery for the first 6 months was the first choice. After 3 months very slight signs of reinnervation appeared at the zygomatic branch. Within 1 year satisfactory reinnervation developed, with only mild synkinesias and some persistent weakness at the frontal muscle, but easy complete eye closure (**e**) and adequate mouth angle control (**f**)

type with nerve recovery starting after 3 months (Fig. 2). Persistent, complete paralysis for 6–10 months requires local exploration and reconstruction.

The facial nerve is first searched at its exit from the stylomastoid foramen. After mobilization of the sternocleido-mastoid muscle and the digastric muscle the styloid process is identified where the facial nerve must be found.

In the case of traumatic destruction of this area, exposure of the nerve at the intratemporal course may become necessary. A small mastoidotomy or mastoidectomy is usually enough to find the healthy proximal part of the nerve.

Next the nerve is to be identified at its extracranial course, at best before its passage through the parotid gland. As soon as the parotid gland is mobilized from the sternocleido-mastoid muscle, the facial nerve as a single stump or two major branches is identified. The proximal intratemporal and the distal extracranial segments are bridged by a transplant for an intratemporal-extracranial reconstruction.

Recovery After Facial Nerve Reconstruction. First signs may be observed after 6–12 months. Within 1–2 years complete eye closure is achieved by 70%–77% of patients (House-Brackmann grade III). Incomplete but evident eye closure and significant mouth control are documented in 18%–29% (House-Brackmann Grade IV). The degree of forceful eye closure and of preserved symmetry on movement depends largely on the timing of the intervention; patients with less favorable results had suffered from long-standing paralysis before they received a nerve reconstruction.

Cochlear Nerve

Causes of cochlear nerve lesions are temporal bone fractures with lesions to the vestibular system, to the inner ear with secondary severe loss of hair cells, ganglion cells, and other supporting cells in the inner ear or with occasional labyrinthitis ossificans. In rare cases of bilateral transverse temporal fractures bilateral loss of audiovestibular function may result [45].

Indication of unilateral cochlear implant is set after MRI [37] and electrical promontory test. In this way the patients with traumatic rupture or secondary scarring and degeneration of the cochlear nerve can be excluded and differentiated from those with a viable cochlear nerve who will profit from a cochlear implant.

Surgery and postoperative rehabilitation program need to be performed by an experienced otorhinolaryngological team [18, 22, 44, 49, 61, 62, 67, 68].

Caudal Cranial Nerves

The caudal cranial nerves can loose their function in severe head traumas with brainstem lesions [25], craniocervical lesions with atlas fracture [27], and at craniocervical penetrating injuries affecting the soft tissues of the neck.

Diagnosis of nuclear caudal nerve lesions is made clinically after recovery from the acute trauma phase, when the patient may show a combination of dysphagia, dysarthria, and weak or hoarse voice. The treatment is conservative and symptomatic; in the early period it aims at prevention of aspiration and later at strengthening of the remnant functions.

Accessory Nerve

Often these lesions occur in polytraumatized patients with combined head and plexus lesions [3]; the accessory lesion may be a consequence of traction trauma, local hit and hemorrhage, or penetrating sharp lesions of the soft tissue. Avellis syndrome is a rare condition occurring in association with infarction of the medulla oblongata sometimes after trauma [34], which usually shows sufficient spontaneous recovery.

Diagnosis of an extracranial lesion of the accessory nerve is evident with trapezius muscle paralysis. The ability to lift the arm over the horizontal plane is lost; this prevents the patient from carrying out many normal day activities and leads to fatigue and sometimes pain.

The indication for surgery is given in all cases of complete palsies as early as possible. Surgery is at first directed towards identification of the proximal nerve segment; the preparation must start proximal to the lesion, at distance from the scar, usually at the posterior border of the sternocleido-mastoid muscle.

In the case of continuity microscopic neurolysis is useful to enable reliable recovery. With neuromatous change this segment should be resected and treated by a sural grafting. If there is discontinuity, the distal nerve stump(s) may be identified at the anterior medial margin of the trapezius muscle; nerve transplantation is the method of choice.

Hypoglossal Nerve

The nerve is endangered in craniocervical traumas with lacerations or direct penetrating injuries to the anterior soft tissues of the neck [33]. In a large series of hypoglossal nerve lesions 10 % were reported to be traumatic in origin, namely due to gunshot wounds. Serious carotid artery lesions may be combined with lesions of the hypoglossal and possibly other caudal nerves. The nerve may also be lesioned secondarily during the management of bleeding vessels. Extremely rare are bilateral hypoglossal lesions in complex head injuries, due to traction injury to both nerves at the base of the skull, possibly on the base of some skull base malformation [31].

Diagnosis is made clinically on deviation of the tongue, blurred speech, difficulty on chewing and swallowing, and atrophy within the first weeks.

The indication for surgery is often given in the acute trauma phase because of the necessity to reconstruct the carotid artery or other lesions of the neck organs. Surgery takes the route to the nerve under the sternocleido-mastoid and the digastric muscles. If the nerve endings can be identified, reconstruction is performed by microsurgical principles.

Principles of Postsurgical Nerve Rehabilitation

The postsurgical program after nerve reconstruction consists of a regular clinical follow-up and physiotherapeutic management:

At outpatient controls every 3–6 months the neurological status and an actual electromyography are evaluated until some reinnervation is documented. Furthermore, the physiotherapeutic exercises performed by the patient are inquired and modified for best adaptation to the actual degree of recovery; especially, exercises for weaker parts of the face or for suppressing synkinesias are explained.

The following is a brief summary of facial physiotherapy instructions [56]:

- A physiotherapy program for at least 3 years consists of daily individual exercises carried out six times for 5–10 min; during the first 1–2 years the patient is accompanied by a specialized physiotherapist during two to three weekly sessions.
- Each exercise consists of the trial of an active movement and thereafter of a massage in the requested direction:
  Lifting eyebrows without any help and striking eyebrows up with the fingertips
  Frowning and pushing eyebrows together
  Closing eyes and sliding down eyelids
  Wrinkling the nose and pushing cheeks together
  Blowing the cheeks and holding the mouth angles tight
  Forming a small "O" with the lips and pushing the mouth angles together
  Smiling and pulling mouth angles apart
  Smiling strongly and pushing the healthy side towards the midline to facilitate some action on the sick side
- If eye closure is especially weak, eye closure is combined with strong biting until eye closure becomes complete. Then the patient tries very slowly to relax the masseter muscles while imaging a closed eye; after complete relaxation the eyes are opened. This whole sequence is repeated three to five times. The same exercise is helpful in reducing synkinesias between eye closure and mouth angle.
- If eye closure is weak in hypoglossal-facial combination, a similar exercise is performed. The eye is closed and supported by pressing the tongue against the teeth; the latter is then very slowly loosened while the eye is tried and imagined to be closed. Within some weeks to months independent eye closure without any tongue movement becomes possible.
- In case of a weak mouth angle the healthy side is pushed towards the midline and fixed with the fingertips; now the sick mouth angle can be trained more easily.
- Any electrical stimulation of nerves or muscles must be avoided in order to minimize the development of contractures.

Clinical Guidelines: Summary for Quick Reference

In the *acute phase*, in the comatose patient quick inspection of head, neck, and face, and is necessary to detect relevant cranial nerve lesions early:

- Ocular hematoma
- Anisocoria
- Irritability at the trigeminal root exit zones
- Retroauricular mastoid hematoma
- Otorrhea, rhinorrhea
- Facial asymmetry

Further precise inspection of bone window CT confirms clinical suspicion:

- Frontal base fracture, involving cribriform plate, ethmoid sinus
- Frontal base fracture, involving optic canal
- Orbital base/maxillary roof fracture
- Maxillary/mandibular fractures close to nerve foramina
- Sphenoid fractures involving the orbital fissure, foramen rotundum, foramen ovale
- Temporal bone fractures involving the internal auditory canal, the cochlea, the semicircular canals
- Posterior fossa fractures involving the jugular foramen, foramen magnum
- Craniocervical instabilities

In the *subacute phase*, after emergency hematoma evacuation and/or cervical stabilization, in the unconscious or noncooperative patient, again, inspection is useful:

- Anisocoria, development of primary or secondary
- Irritability at the trigeminal root exit zones
- Ocular movements on doll's head maneuver
- Otorrhea, rhinorrhea
- Facial asymmetry
- Reaction to acoustic stimuli
- Oropharynx asymmetry

In the *intermediate phase*, in the conscious, (partially) cooperative patient examination must focus on:

- Visual acuity and fields
- Ocular movements
- Trigeminal function (sensory and motor) and irritability
- Facial innervation
- Acoustic function
- Oropharynx symmetry, fluid swallowing, voice strength

On suspicion of a motoric palsy of a cranial nerve EMG is useful after 2 weeks. Photodocumentation of the palsy is useful. Physiotherapy is started.

In complex craniofacial lesions an interdisciplinary treatment is planned involving neurosurgical, ophthalmological, otorhinolaryngological, and maxillofacial teams.

Summary and Conclusions

In mild to severe head injury:

1. The cranial nerve most urgently to be examined and treated is the optic nerve. In case of suspicion of serious optic nerve compression high-dose steroids and immediate nerve decompression are indicated within the first 6 h. Only if some function is preserved before surgery may improvement be anticipated, to an unknown degree.

2. The cranial nerve most frequently affected is the facial nerve. In cases of persistent paralysis exploration and microsurgical nerve reconstruction must be performed within the first 12 months. During the waiting period physiotherapy and presentation to a center for skull base lesions and nerve reconstruction are important. A nerve reconstructive procedure is by far superior to any plastic interventions.

3. The sensory nerve most important to be reconstructed within the first months is the ophthalmic nerve. A comparison of devastating lesions with keratitis neuroparalytica and its successful prevention by nerve reconstruction gives this clear, although rare, indication.

4. A rare but most dangerous lesion involves caudal cranial nerve palsies, due to medullary hematomas with involvement of several brainstem nuclei. The complex disturbances predispose to aspiration and can be prevented only by early detection, possibly temporary tracheostomy, and special rehabilitation.

5. The least frequent lesion is bilateral deafness. In view of the satisfying results with cochlear implants this indication should be tested and offered to the patient.

Fortunately, focal cranial nerve lesions in general do not constitute the life-threatening component in head injuries. Still, their early detection and adequate treatment are significant determinants for the long-term life quality of patients who are rescued on the basis of the optimized trauma program.

References

1. Arai H, Sato K, Yanai A (1995) Hemihypoglossal-facial nerve anastomosis in treating uni-
    lateral facial palsy after acoustic neurinoma resection. J Neurosurg 82(1): 51–54
2. Balcer LJ, Galetta SL, Bagley LJ, Pakola SJ (1996) Localization of traumatic oculomotor
    nerve palsy to the midbrain exit site by magnetic resonance imaging. Am J Ophthalmol
    122(3): 437–439
3. Berry H, MacDonald EA, Mrazek AC (1991) Accessory nerve palsy: a review of 23 cases.
    Can J Neurol Sci 18(3): 337–341

4. Blum M, Tetz MR, Greiner C, Voelcker HE (1996) Treatment of traumatic cataracts. J Cataract Refract Surg 22(3): 342–346
5. Braam MJ, Nicolai JP (1993) Axonal regeneration rate through cross-face nerve grafts. Microsurgery 14(9): 589–591
6. Bunnell S (1927) Suture of the facial nerve within the temporal bone. With a report of the first successful case. Surg Gynecol Obstet 45: 7–12
7. Cardwell EP (1938) Direct implantation of free nerve grafts between facial muscularure and facial trunc. Arch Otolaryng 27: 469–471
8. Coiffier T, Cabanes J, Visot A, Dupuy M, Freche C, Chabolle F (1995) Le traitement endonasal des rhinorrheescerebro-spinales iatrogenes ou spontanees de l'etage anterieur de la base ducrane. Ann Otolaryngol Chir Cervicofac 112(8): 367–373
9. Conley J, Baker DCI (1978) The surgical treatment of extratemporal facial paralysis: an overview. Head Neck Surg 1(1): 12–23
10. Conley JJ (1955) Facial nerve grafting in treatment of parotid gland tumors. Arch Surg 70: 359–366
11. Conley JJ (1961) Facial nerve grafting. Arch Otolaryngol 73: 322–327
12. Cook MW, Levin LA, Joseph MP, Pinczower EF (1996) Traumatic optic neuropathy. Ameta-analysis. Arch Otolaryngol Head Neck Surg 122(4): 389–392
13. Cornelius CP, Ehrenfeld M, Wiethölter H (1994) Late results after reconstruction of the sensory branches of the mandibular nerve. In: Samii M (ed) Skull base surgery. Karger Basel, pp 639–646
14. Cornelius CP, Altenmuiler E, Ehrenfeld M (1996) The use of flash visual evoked potentials in the early diagnosis of suspected optic nerve lesions due to craniofacial trauma. J Craniomaxillofac Surg 24(1): 1–11
15. Cusimano MD, Sekhar L (1994) Partial hypoglossal to facial nerve anastomosis for reinnervation of the paralyzed face in patients with lower cranial nervepalsies: technical note. Neurosurgery 35(3): 532–533 (discussion 533–534)
16. Deruty R, Guyotat J, Mottolese C (1988) Partial recovery of the oculomotor nerve after section and repair during the excision of a tumor. Neurochirurgie 34: 287–292
17. Desaulty A, Nguyen KT, Lansiaux V, Evrard I (1994) Les sections du nerf facial. A propos de 40 observations. Ann Otolaryngol Chir Cervicofac 111(7): 377–384
18. Dillier N, Frolich T, Kompis M, Bogli H, Lai WK (1993) Digital signal processing (DSP) applications for multiband loudness correction digital hearing aids and cochlear implants. J Rehabil Res Dev 30(1): 95–109
19. Dott NM (1958) Facial paralysis. Restitution by extrapetrous nerve graft. Proc R Soc Med 51: 900–902
20. Draf W, Samii M (1982) Intracranial-intratemporal anastomosis of the facial nerve after cerebellopontine angle tumor surgery. In: Graham MD, House WF (eds) Disorders of the facial nerve. Raven, New York, pp 441–449
21. Favre JJ, Chaffanjon P, Passagia JG, Chirossel JP (1995) Blood supply of the olfactory nerve. Meningeal relationships and surgical relevance. Surg Radiol Anat 17(2): 133–138
22. Gantz BJ, Woodworth GG, Knutson JF, Abbas PJ, Tyler RS (1993) Multivariate predictors of audiological success with multichannel cochlear implants. Ann Otol Rhinol Laryngol 102(12): 909–916
23. Grimson BS, Ross MJ, Tyson G (1984) Return of function after intracranial resuture of the trochlear nerve. Case report. J Neurosurg 61: 191–192
24. Guerrero AL, Onzain JI, Martin JA, Blanco A, Moreta JA (1996) Lesion aislada del nucleo de Edinger-Westphal enrelacion topografica con hematoma mesencefalico postraumatico. Rev Neurol 24(132): 982–984
25. Haig AJ, Ho KC, Ludwig G (1996) Clinical, physiologic, and pathologic evidence for vagus dysfunction in a case of traumatic brain injury. J Trauma 40(3): 441–444
26. Hausamen JE, Samii M, Schmidseder R (1973) Repair of the mandibular nerve by means of autologous nerve grafting after resection of the lower jaw. J Maxillofac Surg 1: 74
27. Henche HR, Lucking CH, Schumacher M (1994) Atlasfrakturen mit Parese kaudaler Hirnnerven. Eine Fallbeschreibung. Z Orthop Ihre Grenzgeb 132(5): 394–398
28. Hickham MJ, Cote DN (1995) Temporal bone fractures. J La State Med Soc 147(12): 527–530

29. House JW, Brackmann DE (1985) Facial nerve grading system. Otolaryngol Head Neck Surg 93: 146–147
30. Jääskeläinen J, Pyykkö I, Blomstedt G, Porras M, Palva T, Troupp H (1990) Functional results of facial nerve suture after removal of acoustic neurinoma: analysis of 25 cases. Neurosurgery 27: 408–411
31. Kacker A, Komisar A, Kakani RS, Reich E, Rothman L (1995) Tongue paralysis following head trauma. J Laryngol Otol 109(8): 770–771
32. Kanzaki J, Kunihiro T, O-Uchi T, Ogawa K, Shiobara R, Toya S (1991) Intracranial reconstruction of the facial nerve. Clinical observation. Acta Otolaryngol Suppl (Stockh) 487: 85–90
33. Keane JR (1996) Twelfth-nerve palsy. Analysis of 100 cases. Arch Neurol 53(6): 561–566
34. Kitanaka C, Sugaya M, Yamada H (1992) Avellis syndrome after minor head trauma: report of two cases. Surg Neurol 37(3): 236–239
35. Klimek L, Laborde G, Mosges R, Wenzel M (1993) Ein neues Verfahren zur Entfernungvon Fremdkopern im Kopfbereich. Unfallchirurg 96(4): 213–216
36. Koerte W (1903) Ein Fall von Nervenpfropfung: des Nervus facialis auf den Nervushypoglossus. Dtsch Med. Wochenschr 29: 293–295
37. Kumakawa K, Takeda H, Mutoh N, Miyakawa K, Yukawa K, Funasaka S (1992) [Image analysis of the inner ear with CT and MR imaging: pre-operative assessment for cochlear implant surgery]. Nippon Jibiinkoka Gakkai Kaiho 95(6): 817–824
38. Kunihiro T, Kanzaki J, O-Uchi T (1991) Hypoglossal-facial nerve anastomosis. Clinical observation. Acta Otolaryngol Suppl (Stockh) 487: 80–84
39. Lalak NJ, Farmer E (1996) Traumatic pseudoaneurysm of the superficial temporal artery associated with facial nerve palsy. J Cardiovasc Surg (Torino) 37(2): 119–123
40. Lanzino G, Sekhar LN, Sen CN, Pomonis S (1994) Reconstruction of cranial nerves III through VI during cavernous sinus surgery. In Samii M (ed) Skull Base Surgery. Karger Basel, pp 477–481
41. Matern G, Matthias C, Mrowinski D (1995) Olfaktorisch evozierte Potentiale (OEP) und Contingent NegativeVariation (CNV) bei der Begutachtung von Riechstörungen. Laryngorhinootologie 74(2): 118–121
42. Maxwell JH (1951) Extratemporal repair of the facial nerve. Ann Otology 60: 1114–1133
43. Maxwell JH (1954) Repair of the facial nerve after facial lacerations. Trans Am Acad Ophthal Otolaryngol 58: 733–740
44. Mens LH, Oostendorp T, van den Broek P (1994) Identifying electrode failures with cochlear implant generated surface potentials. Ear Hear 15(4): 330–338
45. Morgan W, Coker NJ, Jenkins HA (1994) Histopathology of temporal bone fractures: implications for cochlear implantation. Laryngoscope 104(4): 426–432
46. Nayak SR, Kirtane MV, Ingle MV (1991) Transethmoid decompression of the optic nerve in head injuries: an update. J Laryngol Otol 105(3): 205–206
47. O'Brien BM, Franklin JD, Morrison WA (1980) Cross-facial nerve grafts and microneurovascular free muscle transfer for long established facial palsy. Br J Plast Surg 33(2): 202–215
48. Pluchino F, Fornari M, Luccarelli G (1986) Intracranial repair of interrupted facial nerve in course of operation for acoustic neurinoma by microsurgical technique. Acta Neurochir 79: 87–93
49. Ponton CW, Don M, Waring MD, Eggermont JJ, Masuda A (1993) Spatio-temporal source-modeling of evoked potentials to acoustic and cochlear implant stimulation. Electroencephalogr Clin Neurophysiol 88(6): 478-4-93
50. Radtke J, Bremerich A, Machtens E (1996) Thermografische Quantifizierung sensibler und sympathischer Nervenläsionen bei Mandibulafrakturen – ein prognostisches Kriterium? Fortschr Kiefer Gesichtschir 41: 176–180
51. Samii M (1972) Autologe Nerventransplantation im Trigeminusbereich. Med Mitt (Melsungen) 46: 189
52. Samii M (1979) Operative treatment of cerebellopontine angle tumors with special consideration of the facial and acoustic nerve. Adv Neurosurg 7: 138–145
53. Samii M (1980) Nerves of the head and neck. In: Omer GE, Spinner M (eds) Management of peripheral nerve problems. Saunders, Philadelphia, pp 507–547
54. Samii M (1981) Preservation and reconstruction of the facial nerve in thecerebellopontine

angle. In: Samii M, Jannetta P (eds) The cranial nerves. Springer, Berlin Heidelberg New York, pp 438-450

55. Samii M, Matthies C (1994) Indication, technique and results of facial nerve reconstruction. Acta Neurochir 130: 125-139
56. Samii M, Matthies C (1997) Management of vestibular schwannomas (acoustic neuromas). VII. The facial nerve: preservation and restitution offunction. Neurosurgery 40 (in print)
57. Samii M, Wallenborn R (1972) Tierexperimentelle Untersuchungen über den Einfluß der Spannung auf den Regenerationserfolg nach Nervennaht. Acta Neurochir 27: 87-110
58. Samii M, Turel KE, Penkert G (1985) Management of seventh and eighth nerve involvement by cerebellopontine angle tumors. Clin Neurosurg 32: 242-272
59. Scaramella L (1971) L'anastomosi tra i due nervi facciali. Arch Ital Otol 82: 207-215
60. Sekhar LN, Lanzino G, Sen CN, Pomonis S (1992) Reconstruction of the third through sixth cranial nerves during cavernous sinus surgery. J Neurosurg 76(6): 935-943
61. Shannon RV (1993) Quantitative comparison of electrically and acoustically evoked auditory perception: implications for the location of perceptual mechanisms. Prog Brain Res 97: 261-269
62. Shepherd RK, Hatsushika S, Clark GM (1993) Electrical stimulation of the auditory nerve: the effect of electrode position on neural excitation. Hear Res 66(1): 108-120
63. Simo R, Jones NS (1996) Extratemporal facial nerve paralysis after blunt trauma. J Trauma 40(2): 306-307
64. Smith JW (1971) A new technique of facial reanimation. In: Transaction fifth international congress of plastic and reconstructive surgery. Butterworths, Melbourne, pp 83-84
65. Stephanian E, Sekhar LN, Janecka IP, Hirsch B (1992) Facial nerve repair by interposition nerve graft: results in 22 patients. Neurosurgery 31(1): 73-76 (discussion 77)
66. Tielsch JM (1996) The epidemiology and control of open angle glaucoma: a population-based perspective. Annu Rev Public Health 17: 121-136
67. Tykocinski M, Shepherd RK, Clark GM (1995) Reduction in excitability of the auditory nerve following electrical stimulation at high stimulus rates. Heart Res 88(1-2): 124-142
68. Weiss MR (1993) Effects of noise and noise reduction processing on the operation of the nucleus-22 cochlear implant processor. J Rehabil Res Dev 30(1): 117-128

15 Neurological, Neurophysiological Syndromes and Cognitive Disorders in Brain-Injured Patients: Epidemiology, Diagnosis, and Therapeutic Advances

W. Gobiet

I. Introduction

Following severe head injury (SHT) cerebral function in spite of consciousness, motoric and cognitive ability cannot be restored without special measures. Vigorous treatment are required to achieve the best outcome for the patient. In order to make full use of the remaining functional capacity of the brain the process of rehabilitation must begin in the acute phase of treatment and continue without a break in the rehabilitation center. The complexity and the interrelated nature of the various lesions necessitate a comprehensive and well thought out plan of management comprising therapeutic, diagnostic, and social elements. Such a concept in turn requires a specially equipped and staffed hospital, and in this way neurotraumatological rehabilitation has developed into an independent discipline [3, 7].

Although almost all types of acute functional disturbances of the central nervous system share the leading symptom of impaired consciousness, head injury patients differ in age, concomitant conditions, and goals of rehabilitation from those with other disease of the CNS. Head injury patients tend to be substantially younger, often still at school or just beginning their working lives. They may still be living with their parents or just have started a family. From the very beginning the treatment must therefore aim at educational or occupational reintegration [4].

Principles of Therapy

Although the recovery from acute brain damage bears some similarity to the stages of development that a child goes through, there are in fact profound differences. The acutely brain-damaged patient had acquired and stored previous intellectual, cognitive, and social experiences and does not have to learn completely from the beginning. Isolated therapeutic approaches generally prove inappropriate for head-injured patient because they are generally designed for use in patients with congenital disorders. Moreover, many of the so-called deficit-oriented therapeutic methods designed to improve motor function often do not achieve the desired goal because they suppress the patient's often minimal voluntary movements, which are important for the patient as a means of expression (orofacial stimulation, basal stimulation, tactile-kinesthetic concept). Experience in more than 2000 cases has shown the value of a complex integrative and learning-centered concept of therapy. The basic principle is early mobilization, the patient's vegetative condition allowing. The patient is stimulated via all channels of sensory perception to elicit active reactions. All reactions are noted and incorporated into initially simple and basic and later more complex answers. The combined and simultaneous stimulation of all senses achieves as great an arousal stimulus as possible, the loss or impairment of one perception being compensated. Normally no passive or isolated procedures should take place without appropriate motor, auditory, and visual support. From the early stage the goal of therapy consists in reactivation of pretraumatic capabilities.

When deciding the appropriate therapy the following points must be observed:

- There are complex deficits where partial losses of function cannot immediately be defined.
- Isolated therapeutic approaches are normally not appropriate because they are designed specifically for use in defined impairment (mostly congential deficits).
- The treatment should be active and didactically constructed following pedagogic principles.
- Falling back on previous knowledge (activation of stored structures) improves the patient's state of alertness and permits rapid restoration of the damaged intellectual cognitive and motoric functions.
- The treatment should combine as wide a range as possible of the impaired and preserved capabilities.
- All of the patient's perception must be stimulated.
- The mode of therapy should motivate the patient.
- The therapist must constantly be able to check grade and possibility of restored functions in order to recognize any progress and modify the treatment in any way necessary.

Observance of these rules has led to the development of a complex integrative and learning-centered concept of treatment for patients with SHT. The goal is reactivation of the disturbed intellectual, cognitive, behavioral and motor functions as rapidly as possible in order to achieve social, occupational and educational reintegration. We term our approach "active directed adapted multisensory stimulation" (ADAMS).

Early Rehabilitation During Acute Treatment

The acute care of head injury patients is a complex matter and is therefore possible only in fully and specially equipped centers. Head injury is accompanied in 70%–80% of cases by other serious injuries, and even today the primary mortality rate is 30%–50%. Close interdisciplinary cooperation can assure optimal acute therapy and prevent secondary complications.

In the forefront are neuromonitoring and the associated therapeutic measures: computed tomography and magnetic resonance imaging – with detailed clinical follow-up, for example, the extended Glasgow Coma System, measurement of intracranial pressure, including computer analysis; cerebral perfusion pressure and cellular oxygen content, transcranial Doppler ultrasound, and electrophysiology with evoked potentials. It must be stressed, however, that personal experience in the treatment of head injuries remains crucial in achieving a successful outcome [8, 12].

In this phase patients show profound impairment of consciousness, with defective or absent brainstem protective reflexes and pathological patterns of posture and movement, vegetative disorders with changes in cardiac rhythm and blood pressure, dramatic variations in metabolism and body temperature, motor dysfunctions as central and peripheral paralyses, and partial or total loss of intellectual and cognitive functions. The majority of patients present a transitory apallic syndrome of variable duration (vegetative state, VS)

In the acute phase medical considerations are central. It is absolutely essential, however, that rehabilitative treatment is initiated without delay, principally by the nursing staff, physicians, physiotherapists, and occupational therapists in the intensive care unit (ICU). The principal components of rehabilitative treatment in the acute phase are sensomotoric activation to raise the patient's level of consciousness and restore the abilities to react, mobilization into a wheelchair, prevention of atrophy and contractures, mitigation of pathological startle and postural reflexes, and facilitation of voluntary movements combined with first steps in activities of daily life (ADL). Normally every step in the patient's care incorporates an element of rehabilitation and activation. Whenever the patient is treated, the member of staff involved must explain, demonstrate, and comment upon the measures while maintaining eye contact, even if it is thought the patient cannot understand the information.

Mobilization of the patient is a important component of the overall activation program. The observation that nearly all patients are much more alert when sitting than when lying down can be confirmed by electrophysiological investigation. In addition, the sitting position facilitates regression of the pathological postural and startle reflexes.

Important for the prevention of atrophy and contractures are appropriate positioning in bed or in wheelchair. There are no general rules: the best position must be established in each individual case. In addition, the patient should undergo several sessions of physiotherapy every day, mobilizing the joints in their principal directions of motion, starting from a spasticity-inhibiting position. These exercises can be carried out, in addition, by nursing staff or even by the patient's relatives. Basic knowledge of physiotherapeutic treatment procedures is helpful. The patient's residual voluntary movements must be recognized and built upon. Events such as bed making, washing, and feeding can be used to improve the patient's voluntary movement and develop motor function. The notion that active or passive movement of the joints in semiconscious or unconscious patients induces calcification has not been confirmed. In addition, antispasmodic medication is necessary. Continuous intrathecal infusion of baclofen or injection of botulinus toxin has proved effective. The development of contractures can be prevented in many cases by orthopedic shoes or by the use of appropriate splints or timely application of an encircling plaster cast.

Other rehabilitatory approaches in the acute phase can be grouped asADL: first exercises in eating, swallowing, or sanitary procedure, structuring of the day by regular meal times or visits to promote disturbed orientation and memory.

The most important task of the relatives is to provide emotional support for the patient by keeping him up to date with family and friends and by giving him personal attention. They should also help to make sure he always performs his life training exercises. When the patient's condition allows, drives outside the ICU are important as external stimuli. It must not be forgotten, however, that the relatives are themselves under abnormal and high emotional stress. Under no circumstances may they be enrolled as substitute nurses or cotherapists.

Treatment in the Rehabilitation Center

Early Rehabilitation

Transfer to a rehabilitation center appropriate to the patient's needs should take place as soon as possible. At this time the patient presents a marked organic brain syndrome, deep or moderate coma, dysfunction in vegetative regulation, and pathological motoric reflexes. Tracheal and gastric tubes and urinary catheter are still in place, and there are load-bearing or non-load-bearing fractures as well as concomitant internal medical and urological problems. The patient either still has an apallic syndrome (VS) or is in the early remission phase. Some patients present severe transitory psychotic syndromes.

The patient's clinical condition necessitates continuation of intensive care. Thus the center must offer an intensive care unit and observation ward with physicians and nurses experienced in neurotraumatology, intensive care, and rehabilitation (early rehabilitation unit, ERU). The laboratory and neuroradiology facilities must be of a correspondingly high standard, and specialists in trauma surgery, internal medicine, ophthalmology, ENT, maxillofacial surgery and neurosurgery must be available for consultation.

The treatment concept demands close coordination of intensive care and therapeutic measures to improve consciousness, intellectual, cognitive and motor functions. As mentioned, however, management depends on the underlying diagnosis. Head-injured patients must be distinguished from those who have suffered other disease of CNS in relation to diagnosis localization, risk factors, and age [7, 11].

In summary, the basic goals of "ADAMS" are: improvement of consciousness, attention, perception and reactions, facilitation of intellectual, cognitive and motor functions, and enhancement of verbal expression, behavior, and interaction in groups. This is the task of an interdisciplinary team.

The *nursing staff*, in addition to basic care, play an important part in activating therapy as ADL, mobilization and voluntary movement, speech facilitation, orientation, behavior, and motivation.

Physiotherapy combats the often massively abnormal postural and startling reflexes. Conservative corrective treatment such as splints, insoles, encircling plaster casts and ice are used in addition to antispasmodic medication by pump infusion of baclofen or botulinus toxin. The goal is free joint movement with facilitation of voluntary motor function and increasing mobilization.

Occupational therapy also includes functional training to restore motor function in the upper and lower limbs and the trunk, as well as ADL combined with therapy to improve cognitive functions, perception, and ability to cope with stress.

Neuropedagogical Therapy restores awareness, attentiveness, and intellectual, cognitive, and motor functions by making use of pretraumatic knowledge. Basic perception and activating treatment is soon followed by more abstract tasks with recognition and writing of numbers and letters, building up to more complex interconnected educational tasks. In severely motor-disabled patients computer-supported therapy with specially developed software and keyboard allows intellectual, cognitive, and motoric approaches.

Parallel *speech therapy* starts by concentrating on improving oropharyngeal motor function. With increasing cooperation, specific diagnosis and treatment of the speech and language disorders become possible. In orofacial problems there is considerable overlap with the therapeutic functions of the nursing staff and other therapists.

Neuropsychological diagnosis should ensue as soon as possible, followed by the appropriate training.

The *senior physician* must have experience in neurology, neurosurgery, internal medicine, traumatology, psychiatry, pediatrics, and rehabilitation. He bears ultimate responsibility for all aspects of the medical and therapeutic process. Continuous support from the other medical disciplines mentioned above is essential.

Other forms of treatment such as music therapy or social education can be introduced if the concept allows it.

The patient's *relatives* provide social contacts, supply emotional support encouragement and motivation, and accompany and support the therapeutic process in general.

Termination of the early phase of rehabilitation is reached when the following criteria are fulfilled: mobilization at least into a wheelchair for more then 2 h; stabilization of vegetative functions; presence and utilization of the ability to communicate; the capacity to participate actively several times a day in treatment sessions lasting up from 30 – 60 min; behavioral improvement for therapy in a small group; and a requirement for nursing care not exceeding 4–6 h daily. It must then be decided whether the criteria for transfer to the next rehabilitation program are fulfilled, or whether continuation of therapy cannot be expected to bring any essential further improvement. Treatment lasts between 3 months and 1–2 years, with each individual case being judged [1, 10].

Follow-Up Rehabilitation

The transition from early rehabilitation to the next phase must be carried out in steps. While the patient still shows definite and often severe intellectual, cognitive, motor, and behavioral deficits, he is better able to cooperate, and additional therapeutic approaches such as pedadogous therapy, neuropsychology, and speech therapy can thus be added. Occupational therapy can also be intensified, especially in the fields of housekeeping, woodwork, metalwork, electronics, and EDV. Intensive physiotherapy continues to be important since nearly all patients still show clear impairments of muscle control, coordination, and voluntary movement.

At the end of this phase it must be decided whether the patient can go on to full or partial educational or occupational reintegration or whether retraining is necessary.

Long-time Activating Care

Unfortunately, there are a number of patients (10% – 15%) having lasting mental, behavior, or motoric deficits that leave them unable to live independently. The degree of disability can extend from continued unconsciousness (VS) to marked mental and physical impairments that render the patient helpless. At this point it must be decided whether the patient can return home with the necessary nursing and therapeutic support or is a suitable candidate for so-called activating care in an appropriate institutional setting.

Outcome

Documentation

The most important forms of documentation are: clinical neurological investigations, video documentation, Glasgow Coma Scale (GCS), Koma-Remissions-Scale (KRS), Functional Independent Mensure (FIM), and Disability Rating Scale (DRS), Barthel index. In spite of the severe and combined dysfunctions scoring provides no certain judgement of the patient's real status and the therapeutic process in the early phase. Reliable results come from clinical and therapeutic investigation combined with video documentation. Of the greatest importance is the personal and experience of the entire staff.

Results

Of 2730 patients treated at our institution 84% have been socially reintegrated, i.e., they have reached at least basic independence in ADL. The total duration of treatment is between 3 months and 2 years (mean 7.2 months). The best results have been: Barthel index > 80, GCS > 2, DRS > 2, isolated SHT, substantial defect in CT under 1.5, midbrain syndrome I–II, unconsciousness < 2 weeks, admission in ERU less than 4 weeks after trauma. The poorest results have been: Barthel index < 40, GCS < 3, DRS < 4, deep midbrain syndrome, unconsciousness > 3 weeks, high grades of polytrauma, lacking or insufficient rehabilitation treatment during acute phase (calcification, decubiti, behavior, etc.) [6].

Analysis of the patients treated in our center compared with data from the literature reveals the following factors that complicate early rehabilitation:

When transferred to our ERU 80% of patients present tracheo-pulmonary complications, 60% have decubitus ulcers and joint lesions (atrophy, calcification), about 5% show endocrine dysfunction. Ages under 9 years or over 50 such as polytrauma or previous cardiovascular or endocrinological diseases have a negative influence. These factors can decisively affect the progress and the outcome of early and follow up rehabilitation. Factors with no influence on outcome are urogenital problems (40%) and problems following neurosurgical or trauma surgical intervention (< 5%). Factors whose effect is as yet unclear but certainly have a great influence on outcome include: circumstances of injury, hypoxie, treatment before hospital admission, acute treatment, and particularly diagnosis, surgery and intensive care, neuromonitoring, and the prevention of secondary damage. The patient's pretraumatic psychosocial situation has not proved decisive for outcome, but it is crucial for the type and extent of reintegration. This is also our experience. As stated in the literature, the depth and duration of initial unconsciousness and the type and extent of brainstem damage play an essential part in determining the outcome [7, 13, 14].

Summary

In recent years neurotraumatological rehabilitation has become an independent discipline. Early rehabilitation must start in the ICU and continue without interruption after the patient has been transferred to an specialized head trauma rehabilitation center with ERU. As our results show, introduction of activating and rehabilitatory treatment in the ICU and their continuation after early transfer from the acute hospital to a specialized rehabilitation center significantly improves the outcome. Particularly important are stimulation and activation by the medical and therapeutic staff (ADAMS), early mobilization, prevention of atrophy and contractures, treatment of pathological reflexes, and facilitation of voluntary motor function. A central rote, especially during the intensive phase, is played by life training (ADL) and treatment directed towards awareness, intellectual and cognitive deficits, orientation, and speech facilitation. Regular visits from relatives support and stimulate the patient. Isolated therapeutic approach cannot fulfill the requirements of head-injured patients.

Our active multisensory therapy (ADAMS) offers many advantages but also presents some problems, principally due to the mobilization of a vegetative instable patients with high risk of infection. Further findings of clinical, technical, and laboratory investigations may allow conclusions regarding treatment techniques and prognosis. The treatment of an unconscious patient would benefit enormously if it could be ascertained by technical means which sensory perceptions are damaged or blocked, and whether stimulation could be improved by concentrating on one particular nondisturbed sense. Investigations must also be carried out to establish whether improvement in the initial and clinical care and more effective prevention of secondary complications during the acute phase can improve the outcome. Our experience shows that rehabilitation and outcome are negatively affected by the following factors: depth and duration of unconsciousness, tracheobronchial complications, primary or secondary brainstem damage, extensive and combined polytrauma, inadequate rehabilitation in the acute phase, undue delay between discharge from the acute hospital and admission to the rehabilitation center, and multiple morbidity. Factors that have a positive effect include early and effective emergency treatment, continuous artificial respiration and neuromonitoring, avoidance of surgery for non-life-threatening conditions in the acute phase and initiation of rehabilitative therapy in the intensive phase [2, 5, 7, 9].

Consistent application of the methods described here enables over 80% of patients with SHT to become fully socially reintegrated and to care for themselves. Successful educational or occupational reintegration is possible in over 60% of cases; 14% remain dependent in ADL, and 4% are in VS. These rates are significantly higher than those without rehabilitation.

References

1. Arbeitsgemeinschaft Neurologische/Neurochirurgische Frührehabiliation (1993) Empfehlungen. Bonn, Bad Godeshöhe, Eigenverlag, Neurologisches Rehabilitationszentrum. Phase II. Heft 8
2. Ahmed I (1988) Use of somatosensory evoked responses in the prediction of outcome from coma. Clin Electroencephalogr 2: 78–86
3. Becker DP, Miller JD, Ward JD et al (1977) The outcome from severe head injury with early diagnosis and intensive management. J Neurosurg 47: 491–502
4. Brooks N, McKinlay W, Symington C et al (1987) Return to work within the first seven years of severe head injury. Brain Inj 1: 5–19
5. Caplan ES, Hoyt N (1981) Infection surveillance an control in the severely traumatized patient. Am J Med 70: 638–640
6. Carlsson C-A, von Essen C, Lorfgren J (1968) Factors affecting the clinic course of patients with severe head injuries. J Neurosurg 29: 242–251
7. Gobiet W (1990) Frührehabilitation nach Schädel-Hirn-Trauma. Springer, Berlin, Heidelberg New York

8. Hollyday PO, Kelly DL, Ball M (1982) Normal computed tomograms in acute head injury: correlation of intracranial pressure, ventricular size and outcome. Neurosugery 10(1): 25–28
9. Johnson DA, Roethig-Johnston K, Richards D (1993) Biochemical and physiological parameters of recovery in acute severe head injury: responses to multisensory stimulation. Brain Inj. 7(6): 491–499
10. Pierce JP, Lyle DM, Quine S et al (1990) The effectiveness of coma arousal intervention. Brain Inj 4: 191–197
11. Rader MA, Alston JB, Ellis DW (1989) Sensory stimulation of severely brain-injured patients. Brain Inj 3: 141–147
12. Rappaport M, Leonard J, Portillo SR (1993) Somatosensory evoked potential peak latencies and amplitudes in contralateral and ipsilateral hemispheres in normal and severely traumatized brain-injured subjects. Brain Inj 7(1): 3–13
13. Schalén W, Hansson L, Nordström G, Nordström C-H (1994) Psychosocial outcome 5–8 years after severe traumatic brain lesions and the impact of rehabilitation services. Brain Inj 8(1): 49–64
14. Spivack G, Spettell CM, Ellis DW, Ross SE (1992) Effects of intensity of treatment and length of stay on rehabilitation outcomes Brain Inj 6(5): 419–434

Subject Index

A waves 7
Abducens nerves 125
Accessory nerve 135
Active multisensory therapy (see also ADAMS) 149
ADAMS (Active multisensory therapy) 149
– goals of 146
Airway care 39
Airway management 36
Airway reflexes 36
American Brain Injury Consortia (ABIC) 1
American Association of Neurological Surgeons (AANS) 51
Amyloid percursor protein 27
Analgesia 32
Anticonvulsant medications
– side effects 63
Anticonvulsants 4
Antioxidants 4
Antispasmodic medication 145, 146
Apallic syndrome (VS) 145
APP (Amyloid percursor protein) 27
Arachidonic acid 10
Arterial blood pressure, middle 14
Arterial hypotension 15
Arterial saturation 37
Arterial venous oxygen difference (AVDO$_2$) 90
Autoregulation 91
Autoregulatory function 8
AVDO$_2$ (Arterial venous oxygen difference) 90, 109
Axonal damage 7

B waves 7
Baclofen 145
Barbiturates 2, 3, 58, 94
– therapy 83
Barthel index 147
Basal stimulation 142
Binocular nerve 124
Blood-brain barrier 11, 83

Bone fractures, temporal 126
Botulinus toxin 145
Bradycardia 37
Bradykinin 10
Brain damage 50
– ischemic 109
– secondary 1
– secondary ischemic 20, 99
Brain edema 10
Brain swelling 73
Brain tissue oxygenation 15
Brain tissue oxygen pressure pO$_2$, p(ti)O$_2$ 6, 15, 99, 111
Brain Trauma Foundation 51
Brainstem, avulsion from the 126

C waves 7
Calcium entry blockers 3
Cardiac function 30
Cardiac output 31
Caudal cranial nerves 134
CBF (Cerebral blood flow) 8, 82
CBF measurements (133xenon) 99
Cell swelling 83
Cerebral blood flow 8, 82, 109
– in newborns 89
Cerebral blood volume, intracranial 9
Cerebral hypoperfusion 45
Cerebral hypoxia 109
Cerebral metabolic rate 83
Cerebral metabolic rate for oxygen (CMRO$_2$) 90, 109
Cerebral perfusion pressure (CPP) 6, 54, 57, 144
– maintenance of 61
Cerebral vascular resistance (CVR) 91
Cerebral vasculature 82
Cerebrospinal fluid (CSF) fistula 68
Cerestat 4
Chronic subdural hematoma 73
Clinical guidelines
– traumatic lesions of cranial nerves in head injured patients 137

Closed head injury 19, 20
CMRO$_2$ (Cerebral metabolic rate for oxygen)
    90, 109
CO$_2$ vasoresponsitivity 82
Cochlear nerve 134
Cognitive ability 142
Coma 73
Complications, extracranial 34
Compression of the basal cisterns 56
Contusion 56, 82
Contusional foci, traumatic 22, 23
Corticosteroids 2
CPP (see Cerebral perfusion pressure)
Cranial base 79
Cranial nerves, lesion of 121
Craniotomy
– suboccipital 128
– osteoplastic 73
CSF (see also Cerebrospinal fluid) 11
CT, three dimensional 78
CVR (Cerebral vascular resistance) 91
Cytokines 84

DAI (see also diffuse axonal injury) 8, 19
Damage, mechanic 89
Deficit-oriented therapeutic methods 142
Diffuse axonal injury (DAI) 19, 20, 27
– Morphology 21
Diffuse secondary brain injury 20
– subtypes of diffuse traumatic brain injury 20
Dihydropyridines 3
Direct face traumas 125
Doppler ultrasound, transcranial 144
Dysfunction in vegetative regulation 145

EAA (see also excitatory amino acids) 10
Early rehabilitation unit (ERU) 145
Electromyography 126
Electrophysiology with evoked potentials 144
Embolization, selective 47
Endonasal endoscopy 123
Endoscopic procedures 73
Endovascular therapy 46
Epidural and subdural hemorrhage,
    traumatic 26
Epidural hematoma 70
ERU (see also early rehabilitation unit) 145
État vermolu 24
European Brain Injury Consortium (EBIC) 1
Excitatory amino acids (EAA) 10
Extension synergisms 14
Extracranial complications 34
Extracranial facial nerve lesions 132

Facial nerve 126
– interruption 131
Facial nerve lesions
– extracranial 132

– nuclear 127
Facial nerve paralysis 121
Facio-facial nerve combination 127
Flexion synergisms 14
Follow-up rehabilitation 147
Food 3
Fractures 56, 68
– comminuted 68
– depressed 68, 69
– linear 68
– mandibular 76, 125
– maxillary 125
– panfacial 76
– zygomatic 76
Free oxygen radicals 10

Ganglion Geniculi 131
– lesions 128
GCS (see also Glasgow Coma Scale) 147
GDC (Guglielmi detachable coils) 48
Glasgow Coma Scale (GCS) 6, 147, 30
Gliding contusion 21, 22
Glucocorticoids 63
Glucose metabolism 86
Glutamate 10, 83
Grafting technique 122
Guglielmi detachable coils (GDC) 48
Guidelines, Management of Severe Head
    injury 50, 65
– topics 52

Head injury
– closed 19, 20
– open 19, 26
– pediatric 89
Hematoma 12, 56
– binocular 124
– chronic subdural 26, 73
– epidural 70
– intracerebral 72
– monocular 124
– subdural 71
– traumatic 68
Hemodynamic monitoring 6
Herniation 13
Histamine 10
House-Brackmann Grading 134
Hydrocephalus 12
Hydroxyethyl starch 31
Hydroxyl radicals 84
Hypercarbia 35
Hyperemia 89
Hypertension, intracranial 109
Hyperventilation 15, 58, 61, 84
– therapy 104
Hypocapneic therapy 85
Hypocapnia
– iatrogenic 61

– induced 104
Hypoglossal nerve 135
Hypoglossal-facial combination 127
Hypotension 29, 54
Hypothermia, moderate 83
Hypovolemic shock 29
Hypoxemia 29
Hypoxia, cerebral 109

Iatrogenic hypocapnia 61
ICP (see intracraniel pressure)
– normal value in adults 12
– treatment 52
ICP monitoring 52, 55
ICP through a ventricular catheter 56
Infections, secondary 81
Inflammatory thrombosis of the cavernous
  sinus 125
Infraorbital rim 78
Initial resuscitation 54, 59, 60
Injury, primary 89
Internal rigid fixation 81
Interruption of the facial nerve 131
Intracerebral hematoma 72
Intracerebral hemorrhage, traumatic 24
Intracranial cerebral blood volume 9
Intracranial hypertension 55, 109
Intracranial pressure (ICP) 6, 9, 14, 91, 144
Intracranial-extracranial nerve transplanta-
  tion 122
Intracranial-intratemporal nerve reconstruc-
  tion 122
Intrapontine hemorrhage 126
Intubation 30, 36
Ischemia 83
Ischemic brain damage 109

Jugular venous blood 86
Jugular venous oxygen saturation (SjvO$_2$) 110
Jugular venous sampling 86

Keratitis neuroparalytica 126

Laceration 24, 25
Lazaroids 11
Le Fort midfacial area 76
Lesion of the cranial nerves 121, 125
– olfactory nerve 123
Leukotrienes 10
Lipid peroxidation 11
Long-time activating care 147

Magnetic resonance imaging (MRI) 69
Mandibular arch 78
Mandibular fractures 76, 125
Mannitol 4, 38, 57, 61, 94
MAP (Mean arterial pressure) 99
Maxillary fractures 125

Mean arterial pressure (MAP) 99
Meningitis, delayed 69
Methylacrylate cement 69
Midline shift 56
Mobilization 144
Monitoring, multimodal 112
Monocular hematoma 124
Mortalitiy in children 89
Motoric ability 142
MRI (Magnetic resonance imaging) 69
Multimodal hemodynamic neuromonitoring
  101
Multimodal monitoring 99, 112
Multiorgan failure 29

Near-infrared spectroscopy (NIRS) 110, 113
Nerve decompression 124
Nerve reconstruction 122
Nerve rehabilitation 135
Nerve stumps 122
Neurological assessment 39
Neuromonitoring parameters 14, 99
Neuromonitoring, multimodal
  hemodynamic 14, 99, 101
Neuropedagogical therapy 146
Neuroprotection 19
Neuroprotective drugs 32
Neuropsychological therapy 146
Nimodipine 3
NIRS (Near-infrared spectroscopy) 110,
  113
Nuclear facial nerve lesions 127
Nutritional support 64

Occupational nerve therapy 146
Oculomotor 125
Open head injury 19, 26
Open reduction 81
Operative measures 69
Optic nerve 124
Orbit 124
Orofacial stimulation 142
Osteoplastic craniotomy 73
Outcome 1, 56, 145
– functional 82
Oxygen free radicals 83

Pain management 32
Pain perception 32
Palatal plate 78
Panfacial fractures 76
Pathological motoric reflexes 145
Pediatric head injury 89
– analgetics 92
– antiepileptics 92
– cerebral perfusion pressure 93
– controlled lumbar drainage 95
– decompressive craniectomy 95

– elevation of the head 92
– hyperventilation 93
– intravenous fluids 92
– muscle relaxants 92
– sedatives 92
Persistent cerebrospinal fluid leakage 123
Phase-1 trials 1
Phase-2 trials 1
Phospholipase C 10
Plain skull X-ray 69
Pneumonia 36
Polytraumata 29
Preclinical management 29
Pressure autoregulation 82
Primary injury 89
Prostaglandine G2 (PGG2) 10
Pseudo-aneurysma 46, 126
Psychotic syndromes 145
PtiO$_2$ see Brain tissue oxygen pressure

Quality assessment 40

Regional oxygen saturation (rSO$_2$) 99, 110
Respiratory disturbances 14
Respiratory function 30
Resuscitation 59
– initial 60
Rhinoliquorrhea 81
Ringer's solution 37

Schizogyria 24
Second tier therapy 61
Secondary brain damage 1
Secondary changes 19
Secondary insults 34
Sedation 32, 38
Seizure, prophylaxis in TBI 63
Seizures, posttraumatic 63
Sensomotoric activation 144
Serotonin 10
Serum osmolarity 62
Severe traumatic brain injury 50
Shock 37
Shunt volume 45
SjvO2 (Jugular venous oxygen saturation) 110
Skull base trauma 125
Spasticity-inhibiting position 144
Speech therapy 146
Stable xenon 99
Stretcher 39

Subdural hematoma
– classification of 71
Subdural space 71
Summary for quick reference
– traumatic lesions of cranial nerves in head
  injured patients 137
Superoxide 84
Supraorbital rim 78

Tactile-kinesthetic concept 142
Temporal segment 131
Temporomandibular joint 76
Therapy
– integrative-centered concept of 143
– learning-centered concept of 143
– neuropedagogical 146
– neuropsychological 146
– occupational 146
– speech 146
Tirilazad 4
Transcranial cerebral oximetry 100
Transcranial Doppler ultrasound 144
Transethmoidal approach 124
Trauma systems 54
Trauma-induced vasospasm 9
Traumatic carotid cavernous fistula
– clinic 44
– etiology 45
– therapy 45
– types of carotid artery-cavernous sinus 44
Traumatic pseudoaneurysm 126
Traumatic subarachnoid hemorrhage 3
Trigeminal nerve 125
Trochlear nerve 125
Trolley 39

Vascular reactivity 8
Vasogenic development 10
Vasomotor paralysis 9
Vasopressor 38
Vegetative regulation, dysfunction 145
Vital function 30
Volume replacement 37

Wallerian degeneration 22

X-ray 69

Zygomatic arch 78
Zygomatic fracture 76